Unofficial PTCB Exam Study Guide:

650 Practice Questions with In-Depth Rationales Covers All Four Domain for the Pharmacy Technician Certification Exam

Caldwell Abiodun

Author Introduction

The lead author brings extensive experience in community and institutional pharmacy settings, including medication dispensing, inventory management, sterile and non-sterile compounding, and regulatory compliance. Pharmacy technicians play a critical role in safeguarding patient health by ensuring prescription accuracy, maintaining proper storage conditions, and adhering to strict safety standards. The PTCE® examination evaluates knowledge across essential domains such as medications, federal requirements, patient safety, and order entry and processing. This guide reflects those responsibilities by translating real-world pharmacy operations into structured, exam-focused preparation aligned with the standards established by the Pharmacy Technician Certification Board (PTCB).

Working collaboratively, the contributing team conducted a comprehensive review of the PTCE® content outline to ensure thorough coverage of its key areas. Detailed attention is given to pharmacology fundamentals, drug classifications, dosage calculations, compounding principles, medication safety protocols, and federal pharmacy law. Each chapter integrates conceptual explanations with practical examples reflective of day-to-day pharmacy operations.

Recognizing that many PTCE® candidates are balancing work, coursework, or training programs, this study guide is intentionally structured for clarity and efficiency. Complex drug information and regulatory concepts are presented in organized, accessible language without sacrificing technical accuracy. Practice questions, calculation exercises, and focused review summaries are incorporated to strengthen retention and build exam-day confidence.

Above all, this resource reflects deep respect for the essential role pharmacy technicians play within the healthcare system. Earning PTCE® certification represents more than passing an examination—it signifies professional competence, dedication to patient safety, and a commitment to excellence in pharmacy practice. It is the sincere intention of the author and collaborative team that this guide serves as both a comprehensive pathway to certification success and a strong foundation for continued professional growth.

Table of Content

This study guide is intended solely for educational and informational purposes. While every effort has been made to ensure the accuracy and reliability of the information presented at the time of publication, the publisher and contributors make no representations or warranties, express or implied, regarding completeness, accuracy, or suitability for any specific purpose. Examination content outlines, eligibility requirements, policies, scoring standards, and regulatory guidelines are subject to change at the discretion of the respective certifying or governing organizations. Readers are responsible for verifying the most current information directly with the appropriate official authority.

The content contained in this publication does not constitute legal, financial, medical, or professional advice. It is designed to supplement official materials, formal instruction, and professional training programs—not to replace them. Use of this guide does not guarantee examination success, certification, licensure, employment, or advancement. Individual outcomes will vary based on preparation, experience, and examination conditions.

Disclaimer

Pharmacy Technician Certification Exam® (PTCE®) is a registered trademark of the Pharmacy Technician Certification Board. This publication is an independent study tool and is not affiliated with or endorsed by PTCB .

Chapter 1- Medications: Introduction and Classification

Understanding medications is the cornerstone of pharmacy technician practice. The PTCE® evaluates not only a technician's familiarity with drug names but also the reasoning that guides their use, classification, and potential risks. Each medication represents a combination of **chemical structure, mechanism of action, and therapeutic effect**—three dimensions that inform safe dispensing and patient education.

Medications are broadly organized into **therapeutic classifications**, grouping drugs that achieve similar outcomes. Examples include **antihypertensives**, which lower blood pressure through mechanisms such as vasodilation or diuretic action, and **antimicrobials**, which eliminate pathogens through interference with cell wall synthesis or protein production. Recognizing the therapeutic class allows technicians to identify potential interactions, storage requirements, and substitution equivalencies when generic alternatives are available.

The distinction between **brand** and **generic names** is fundamental. Brand names are proprietary identifiers owned by manufacturers, while generic names reflect the medication's chemical composition and are standardized internationally. Technicians must accurately interpret both names to prevent dispensing errors—particularly in settings where look-alike or sound-alike drugs can pose risk. The PTCE® expects candidates to demonstrate precision when matching a prescription's written order to the correct medication, strength, and dosage form.

A strong command of pharmacologic terminology enables technicians to navigate medication classes confidently, communicate effectively with pharmacists, and ensure patient safety through informed verification.

Mechanisms of Action and Therapeutic Use

A technician's understanding of drug mechanisms enhances their ability to anticipate medication effects and recognize potential complications. **Mechanism of action** describes how a drug produces its intended therapeutic effect—whether by stimulating receptor activity, inhibiting enzyme function, or altering cellular signaling. For instance, **beta-blockers** reduce heart rate by preventing adrenaline from binding to beta-adrenergic receptors, while **proton pump inhibitors** decrease gastric acid secretion by blocking the hydrogen-potassium ATPase enzyme in stomach lining cells.

Knowledge of therapeutic use helps ensure that technicians can identify when a prescribed drug aligns with the patient's diagnosis or reported symptoms. For example, **metformin** is prescribed for type 2 diabetes due to its effect on hepatic glucose production, while **lisinopril**, an ACE inhibitor, treats hypertension by preventing the conversion of angiotensin I to angiotensin II. Recognizing these relationships allows technicians to flag discrepancies that might require pharmacist review.

Equally critical is familiarity with **drug duplication**—when two medications with similar therapeutic outcomes are prescribed concurrently, increasing risk of adverse effects. According to the provided material, technicians should be trained to identify duplications in categories such as pain management, antihypertensive therapy, and central nervous system depressants. Effective medication reconciliation depends on this vigilance.

The PTCE® assesses this domain with questions requiring candidates to apply reasoning rather than rote memorization. For example, understanding why two antihypertensives might interact or how a specific dosage form affects absorption reflects comprehension of clinical context—a core expectation of certification.

Dosage Forms, Routes, and Drug Stability

The **formulation** of a medication determines how it delivers therapeutic effects and influences its handling within the pharmacy. Technicians must know both **dosage forms** and **routes of administration** to ensure safe, appropriate dispensing. Common oral dosage forms include **tablets, capsules, and liquids**, while parenteral forms encompass **injectables, infusions, and reconstituted powders**. Topical, ophthalmic, otic, and transdermal forms serve localized or systemic purposes depending on the absorption characteristics of the active ingredient.

Each route carries specific handling requirements. Injectable medications demand aseptic technique and attention to sterility, whereas oral and topical agents require awareness of contamination prevention and expiration dating. Understanding the purpose behind dosage design—such as **extended-release formulations**—helps technicians avoid substitutions that could alter therapeutic outcomes.

Drug stability is another critical consideration. Factors such as **temperature, light exposure, and moisture** can degrade active ingredients. Insulins, vaccines, and reconstitutable suspensions often require refrigeration and limited shelf life once opened or mixed. Labeling must reflect storage instructions accurately, ensuring the medication maintains its efficacy until the patient's final dose.

Technicians also monitor **beyond-use dates (BUDs)** for compounded or repackaged medications, distinguishing them from manufacturer-assigned expiration dates. The PTCE® expects familiarity with stability parameters as defined in federal and professional standards, particularly for products handled in both sterile and non-sterile environments.

Drug Interactions and Contraindications

Drug interactions are among the most critical areas of pharmacy technician awareness. Interactions occur when the pharmacologic or therapeutic effect of one medication is altered by the presence of another substance—whether a drug, dietary component, or laboratory reagent. The PTCE® expects familiarity with **drug–drug, drug–disease, drug–nutrient, and drug–supplement interactions**, emphasizing the technician's role in prevention and communication.

Drug–drug interactions may lead to reduced efficacy or heightened toxicity. For example, combining **warfarin** with **nonsteroidal anti-inflammatory drugs** increases the risk of bleeding, while **macrolide antibiotics** may elevate serum levels of certain statins, raising the likelihood of muscle toxicity. Similarly, **drug–disease interactions**—such as prescribing a nonselective beta-blocker to an asthmatic patient—can worsen underlying conditions.

Contraindications define situations in which a medication should not be used due to risk outweighing benefit. These may be **absolute**, as with pregnancy exposure to teratogenic drugs like isotretinoin, or **relative**, requiring caution and professional judgment. Technicians contribute to safety by recognizing red-flag conditions noted in patient profiles and alerting the pharmacist when a potential conflict arises.

To manage these risks, technicians should routinely verify active medication profiles, review auxiliary labels, and consult approved reference databases before dispensing. Consistent vigilance minimizes the potential for adverse drug events and ensures adherence to established pharmacy safety protocols.

Adverse Effects, Side Effects, and Allergic Reactions

While side effects are often mild and expected, **adverse drug events (ADEs)** and **allergic reactions** require immediate attention. Side effects typically reflect predictable pharmacologic actions—such as drowsiness from antihistamines—whereas ADEs may result from dosing errors, unexpected sensitivity, or systemic toxicity.

Allergic reactions represent immune-mediated responses to specific drug molecules or their metabolites. Common triggers include **penicillin derivatives**, **sulfa-containing medications**, and certain **anticonvulsants**. Technicians play a vital role in preventing repeated exposure by confirming patient allergy status during intake and maintaining accurate records in the pharmacy information system.

Recognition of **high-alert medications**—those with narrow therapeutic ranges or severe outcome potential—is essential. According to the provided material, this category includes anticoagulants, insulins, opioids, and chemotherapeutic agents. Technicians must apply heightened verification steps, such as double-checking National Drug Code (NDC) numbers and verifying strength and formulation against the original order.

Error prevention in this context depends on a systematic workflow: reading the label three times (when selecting, preparing, and returning the drug), verifying patient identifiers, and ensuring proper counseling is available through the pharmacist. For the PTCE®, candidates should be prepared to identify scenarios where these precautions apply and understand how to respond when discrepancies arise.

Storage, Handling, and Domain 1 Summary

Proper **storage and handling** preserve medication integrity from receipt to administration. Technicians must maintain correct temperature ranges—ambient (20–25°C), refrigerated (2–8°C), and frozen (−20°C)—as stated on manufacturer packaging. Certain medications, such as **insulin**, **vaccines**, and **reconstitutable antibiotics**, degrade rapidly if stored improperly. Others, like **nitroglycerin tablets**, are sensitive to light and moisture and should remain in original containers until use.

Inventory control also involves segregating hazardous and non-hazardous substances, following facility protocols for restricted-access drugs, and ensuring controlled substances are locked and logged per federal requirements. When medications near expiration, technicians must remove and document them appropriately to prevent dispensing errors.

Domain 1 Summary:
The PTCE®'s Medications section tests a candidate's comprehension of pharmacologic principles and real-world application. Success in this area depends on mastery of:

- Generic and brand name equivalence
- Drug classes and mechanisms of action

- Recognition of duplications and contraindications
- Safe handling, storage, and labeling practices

To prepare effectively, candidates should create flashcards by therapeutic class, summarize high-alert drug lists, and routinely practice scenario-based questions involving interactions or dosing errors. Reviewing commonly prescribed medications by indication reinforces retention and enhances accuracy under exam conditions.

Chapter 2- Federal Drug Control Framework

Federal pharmacy regulation establishes the structure through which medications are classified, distributed, and monitored in the United States. These standards exist to ensure **public safety**, **accountability**, and **integrity in pharmaceutical practice**. The PTCE® tests knowledge of major federal laws and agencies governing medication use, including their practical implications in daily pharmacy operations.

The **Food and Drug Administration (FDA)** oversees drug approval, labeling, and post-market surveillance, while the **Drug Enforcement Administration (DEA)** regulates controlled substances under the **Controlled Substances Act (CSA)**. Technicians must understand how these agencies coordinate—FDA evaluating safety and efficacy, DEA enforcing restriction and accountability for abuse-prone medications.

Controlled substances are categorized into **five schedules** based on potential for abuse and accepted medical use:

- **Schedule I (C-I):** No accepted medical use; highest abuse potential (e.g., heroin, LSD).
- **Schedule II (C-II):** High abuse potential, accepted medical use, severe restriction (e.g., morphine, oxycodone).
- **Schedule III (C-III):** Moderate abuse potential (e.g., acetaminophen with codeine).
- **Schedule IV (C-IV):** Low abuse potential (e.g., benzodiazepines).
- **Schedule V (C-V):** Lowest abuse potential; may include limited narcotics in antitussives or antidiarrheals.

Each schedule dictates handling, documentation, and refill restrictions. For example, **C-II prescriptions** cannot be refilled and require a written or electronic order signed by the prescriber. Pharmacy technicians are responsible for verifying DEA numbers, maintaining accurate records, and alerting pharmacists to discrepancies.

Prescription Handling, Labeling, and Disposal

Federal regulations detail how medications—particularly controlled substances—must be **received, stored, dispensed, and disposed of** within a pharmacy. Technicians act as frontline custodians of compliance, ensuring that all procedures align with DEA and FDA expectations.

Upon receipt, controlled substances must be verified against invoices, recorded in perpetual inventory, and stored in a **secure, locked cabinet** or dispersed throughout stock in a manner that deters theft. Inventory logs must be reconciled regularly and retained for at least two years, though some state laws extend this requirement.

Dispensing and labeling requirements mandate that each prescription label include patient and prescriber information, the date filled, drug name, strength, directions for use, and cautionary statements. Controlled substances carry additional labeling such as "Caution: Federal law prohibits the transfer of this drug to any person other than the patient for whom it was prescribed."

Disposal of expired or damaged controlled medications must occur through DEA-authorized **reverse distributors** or take-back programs. Pharmacies must document each transfer or destruction event with DEA Form 41 and maintain records for audit purposes. Technicians must never dispose of controlled substances independently; all actions must be supervised and logged.

Technicians also assist in managing **non-hazardous pharmaceutical waste**, ensuring compliance with Environmental Protection Agency (EPA) standards and preventing contamination of the public water supply. According to provided materials, these steps help maintain patient safety and institutional credibility.

Federal Safety and Compliance Programs

Several federal programs establish systems for monitoring, reporting, and preventing medication misuse or quality defects. Understanding these is essential for PTCE® success and professional competence.

The **Drug Supply Chain Security Act (DSCSA)** requires serialization and traceability of all prescription drugs to prevent counterfeit products from entering distribution. Technicians must ensure that lot numbers and expiration dates are tracked in accordance with DSCSA standards and that any suspicious products are quarantined immediately.

The **Risk Evaluation and Mitigation Strategies (REMS)** program, administered by the FDA, mandates specific safety controls for high-risk medications. Examples include pregnancy prevention programs for isotretinoin or mandatory lab testing for clozapine. Technicians must be aware of which medications fall under REMS requirements and confirm that documentation is complete before dispensing.

Medication recalls are managed through the FDA's recall classification system:

- **Class I:** Serious adverse health consequences or death possible.
- **Class II:** Temporary or medically reversible effects possible.
- **Class III:** Unlikely to cause harm but violate labeling or manufacturing standards.

Technicians are responsible for identifying and removing affected lots, recording actions, and ensuring patients receive replacements or notifications. Timely response to recalls is a regulatory and ethical duty.

Domain 2 Summary:
Federal Requirements test a technician's understanding of legal accountability, from prescription control to waste management. Mastery involves remembering key forms, storage laws, DEA number validation, and recall response.
When presented with scenarios, apply the **"lowest risk, highest compliance"** rule—choose actions that enhance traceability, supervision, and documentation.

FDA Recalls and Product Tracking

The **Food and Drug Administration (FDA)** monitors product quality and safety after approval through ongoing surveillance and consumer reporting. When a drug or medical product is found to be defective or potentially harmful, the FDA issues a **recall**. Understanding recall classifications and technician responsibilities is an essential PTCE® skill.

Recalls fall into three categories:

- **Class I:** Products that may cause serious health consequences or death.
- **Class II:** Products that may cause temporary or medically reversible health problems.
- **Class III:** Products unlikely to cause harm but violate labeling or manufacturing regulations.

Pharmacy technicians must ensure that recalled medications are **immediately removed** from active stock and **segregated** to prevent further dispensing. The lot numbers and expiration dates of affected items should be compared against recall notices distributed by manufacturers, wholesalers, or the FDA. Affected inventory is then returned, documented, or destroyed in accordance with facility policy.

Under the **Drug Supply Chain Security Act (DSCSA)**, pharmacies must maintain product traceability through serial numbers, transaction records, and tracking documents for six years. Technicians ensure compliance by recording the **product identifier**, **lot number**, **expiration date**, and **transaction statement** for each drug shipment received. This system ensures every medication can be traced from manufacturer to dispenser, promoting supply chain integrity and patient safety.

Restricted Programs and Controlled Substance Documentation

Certain medications require special handling under **federal restricted drug programs**, designed to mitigate specific risks. Examples include the **iPLEDGE program** for isotretinoin, which prevents fetal exposure, and **Clozapine REMS**, requiring patient enrollment and lab monitoring due to risk of agranulocytosis. Technicians must verify compliance documentation before dispensing and record confirmations in the pharmacy system.

Controlled substances demand meticulous recordkeeping and verification at every stage of handling. Pharmacies must maintain a **perpetual inventory** for Schedule II medications and separate documentation for other schedules. Required DEA forms include:

- **Form 222:** Ordering or transferring Schedule II substances.
- **Form 41:** Documenting destruction of controlled substances.
- **Form 106:** Reporting loss or theft.

Each entry must include drug name, strength, quantity, date, and signature of authorized personnel. Technicians assist in reconciling inventory counts, ensuring accurate entries, and identifying discrepancies promptly.

Loss or theft of controlled substances must be reported to the DEA within one business day. A copy of Form 106 must also be filed with state authorities when required. In practice, technicians serve as the first line of defense by monitoring daily transaction patterns and reporting any irregularities to the supervising pharmacist.

Proper disposal of **hazardous pharmaceuticals**, such as chemotherapy agents or cytotoxics, is governed by **EPA hazardous waste regulations**. These substances are identified under **P-list** and **U-list** categories, and technicians must segregate waste accordingly to ensure safe removal and environmental protection.

Chapter 3- Foundations of Patient Safety and Quality Assurance

Patient safety lies at the core of pharmacy practice, integrating accuracy, accountability, and ethical duty. The PTCE® devotes a substantial portion of its content to evaluating how technicians contribute to safe medication use. According to the provided material, quality assurance in pharmacy encompasses **error prevention, event reporting, continuous process improvement, and adherence to established protocols**.

A medication error is any preventable event that may cause or lead to inappropriate medication use or patient harm. These events can occur at any stage—prescribing, transcribing, dispensing, or administration. Pharmacy technicians, positioned at the operational heart of these processes, play a critical role in detection and prevention.

Maintaining a **safety-first mindset** begins with environmental awareness. Workstations should be clean, well-lit, and organized to minimize distractions. Each task, from counting tablets to labeling, must follow the "five rights" framework: **right patient, right drug, right dose, right route, right time**.
Even when automated dispensing technology assists in workflow, technicians must verify each selection visually before final pharmacist review.

A well-designed quality assurance program includes **double-check systems**, **barcode verification**, and **standardized labeling procedures**. The ultimate goal is consistency: ensuring that every step of medication handling produces identical results regardless of personnel or shift changes.

High-Alert and Look-Alike/Sound-Alike Medications

Some drugs present greater risk of harm when errors occur. These are designated **high-alert medications** by professional safety organizations and are emphasized in the PTCE® outline. Examples include **insulins, anticoagulants, opioids, chemotherapeutic agents, and concentrated electrolytes**. Due to their narrow therapeutic ranges, even small deviations in dosage or formulation can result in severe outcomes.

Technicians mitigate risk by following precise procedures: storing high-alert medications in separate, clearly labeled sections; applying **Tall Man lettering** (e.g., "hydrOXYzine" vs. "hydrALAZINE") to differentiate look-alike names; and verifying high-alert drugs using barcode technology prior to final pharmacist check. Many pharmacies also use colored shelf tags, warning stickers, or bin dividers to highlight these medications visually.

Look-alike/sound-alike (LASA) medications, another major source of dispensing error, require particular vigilance. Examples include **Celebrex® (celecoxib)** and **Celexa® (citalopram)** or **Zyrtec® (cetirizine)** and **Zyprexa® (olanzapine)**. Confusion may occur during transcription or data entry. Verifying each prescription's indication and dosage form helps prevent LASA-related mistakes.

An important PTCE® concept is **error prevention through system design** rather than individual correction. By creating environments that anticipate human fallibility—such as barcode scanning and separate storage—technicians strengthen safety without relying solely on memory or attention.

Communication and Error Reporting Systems

Accurate communication between technicians, pharmacists, prescribers, and patients forms the backbone of safe medication practice. Miscommunication is a leading cause of medication errors, particularly during prescription intake or handoff. Effective communication relies on **clear documentation**, **active listening**, and **use of standardized abbreviations** consistent with institutional policy. The PTCE® expects candidates to recognize and avoid **error-prone abbreviations** such as "U" for units, "QD" for daily, and trailing or leading zeros that can cause misinterpretation.

When an error or near-miss occurs, reporting it promptly allows corrective action and systemic improvement. Pharmacy quality assurance programs use tools such as:

- **MedWatch** – FDA's voluntary reporting program for adverse events and product issues.
- **VAERS** – Vaccine Adverse Event Reporting System for post-immunization effects.
- **CQI and RCA** – Continuous Quality Improvement and

Event Reporting and Continuous Improvement

Event reporting is an essential feature of any pharmacy safety system. When errors, near-misses, or adverse effects occur, documentation provides the foundation for analysis and future prevention. The PTCE® requires knowledge of **how and why these reports are made**, as well as which agencies oversee specific categories of events.

MedWatch, administered by the FDA, is used for reporting serious adverse drug reactions, product quality defects, and device failures. **VAERS** (Vaccine Adverse Event Reporting System) is jointly operated by the FDA and CDC to track post-immunization reactions. These systems rely on timely submission by healthcare professionals, including pharmacy staff.

Pharmacies also maintain internal **Continuous Quality Improvement (CQI)** programs. Through **Root Cause Analysis (RCA)**, they identify the underlying factors behind errors—such as workflow bottlenecks, ambiguous labeling, or interruptions—and implement procedural changes. CQI focuses on improving systems rather than assigning blame.

Technicians contribute to this culture by documenting incidents objectively and suggesting corrective actions. For example, if multiple counting errors arise with a particular medication, CQI procedures might include adjusting workflow, increasing barcode utilization, or redesigning label placement. By participating in CQI, technicians support measurable, lasting safety enhancements.

Infection Prevention and Compounding Standards

Infection prevention in the pharmacy setting is vital to maintaining sterile product integrity and patient health. The PTCE® emphasizes technician proficiency in **cleaning procedures, hand hygiene, and aseptic handling techniques**.

Before preparing or packaging any medication, technicians must follow the **handwashing protocol** using antimicrobial soap and warm water for a minimum of 30 seconds, ensuring all surfaces of the hands and wrists are scrubbed. Use of gloves, hair covers, masks, and gowns prevents contamination during sterile compounding.

Cleaning and disinfection routines include wiping counting trays and countertops with approved sanitizing agents between uses, avoiding cross-contamination between hazardous and non-hazardous materials. Equipment such as mortars, pestles, and balances should be cleaned immediately after use according to manufacturer guidelines.

Sterile compounding areas must comply with standards similar to those described in professional pharmacy compounding guidelines. These areas are classified by air cleanliness levels (ISO Class 5–8) and require periodic certification. Technicians working in these environments are trained to maintain laminar airflow, perform aseptic manipulations, and minimize particle generation through controlled movements and appropriate garbing.

Adherence to infection control procedures not only protects patients but also reduces occupational exposure risks for pharmacy personnel. Proper documentation of cleaning schedules and environmental monitoring results demonstrates compliance during inspections.

Download Audio file and flashcards

Chapter 4- Overview of Order Entry and Processing

The **Order Entry and Processing** domain evaluates a technician's ability to receive, interpret, and prepare medication orders accurately. This area integrates technical precision with legal and safety compliance. The PTCE® expects candidates to demonstrate mastery of **medical terminology, pharmaceutical calculations, abbreviations, and prescription validation procedures**.

Pharmacy technicians function as the first checkpoint in the medication distribution process. Every order must be reviewed for completeness before it reaches the pharmacist for verification. Essential components include:

- **Patient information:** name, date of birth, address, and allergies.
- **Prescriber details:** name, DEA or license number (if applicable), and signature.
- **Medication specifics:** drug name, strength, dosage form, quantity, and directions for use.

Technicians must verify each element for clarity, ensuring the order follows both **state and federal law**. Ambiguities—such as unclear handwriting, missing directions, or conflicting dosages—must be referred to the pharmacist before processing.

Pharmacy computer systems support order entry by populating standard fields and applying clinical decision support tools, such as **drug–drug interaction alerts**. While these systems enhance safety, human oversight remains critical; automated alerts can be bypassed or misinterpreted if reviewed superficially. The PTCE® emphasizes the technician's responsibility to confirm every field's accuracy before label generation.

Pharmaceutical Calculations and Conversions

Calculation accuracy underpins safe dispensing and is a heavily weighted skill within this domain. The PTCE® assesses arithmetic, algebraic reasoning, and proportional analysis related to medication dosage, compounding, and dilution. Mastery of these skills ensures correct preparation and administration of medications across all practice settings.

Core Calculation Principles:

1. **Ratio and Proportion:**
   a/b=c/d*a*/*b*=*c*/*d* → cross-multiplying to find the unknown quantity.
   Example: If 250 mg corresponds to 5 mL, how many milligrams are in 3 mL?
   250/5=x/3⇒x=150250/5=*x*/3⇒*x*=150 mg.

2. **Dimensional Analysis:**
   A universal conversion approach linking units step by step.
   Example: Convert 1.5 g to mg.
   1.5 g×1000 mg/g=1500 mg1.5 g×1000 mg/g=1500 mg.

3. **Percentage and Dilution Formulas:**
   Used to adjust solution strength.

C1V1=C2V2*C*1*V*1=*C*2*V*2

Example: Prepare 50 mL of a 5% solution using a 10% stock solution:

(10)(x)=(5)(50)⇒x=25(10)(*x*)=(5)(50)⇒*x*=25 mL of stock solution.

4. **Dosage by Weight:**

   Dose=Weight×Dosage rateDose=Weight×Dosage rate.

   Example: Administer 5 mg/kg for a 60 kg patient → 300 mg total.

Technicians must perform all calculations without reliance on external devices unless approved, as on-screen calculators may be provided during testing. Accuracy requires both mathematical proficiency and understanding of context—ensuring units, dosage forms, and patient factors align logically.

Measurement Systems and Accuracy Control

Pharmacy calculations depend on precise measurement systems. The PTCE® focuses on **metric, apothecaries', and household systems**, emphasizing conversions between them.

Common Metric Equivalents:

- 1 g = 1000 mg
- 1 mL = 1 cc
- 1 kg = 2.2 lb

Household Conversions:

- 1 tsp = 5 mL
- 1 tbsp = 15 mL
- 1 fl oz = 30 mL

Accuracy Control Procedures:

- Always verify **significant figures** and avoid rounding until the final step.
- Double-check calculated results against reasonable dosage ranges.
- Conduct **independent verification**: another technician or the pharmacist reviews the same calculation separately before preparation.
- For compounding or reconstitution, record all weights and volumes immediately in the compounding log, ensuring traceability.

Case Example:

A prescription requires 250 mg/5 mL of a liquid antibiotic. The patient's dose is 125 mg. Calculation:

(125mg)/(250mg)×5mL=2.5mL(125*mg*)/(250*mg*)×5*mL*=2.5*mL*.

The technician accurately measures 2.5 mL per dose, confirms the label, and documents the calculation for verification.

Exam Tip:

PTCE® questions in this domain frequently involve multi-step problems. Write out each conversion and verify logic before selecting an answer—speed is valuable, but accuracy is essential. Always confirm that the final unit matches what the question requests.

Understanding Sig Codes and Medical Abbreviations

Interpreting **Sig codes**—standardized prescription abbreviations—is an essential pharmacy technician competency. "Sig" derives from the Latin *signa*, meaning "write" or "label." These codes convey instructions for dosage, frequency, and administration route. While abbreviations improve workflow efficiency, misinterpretation can lead to serious medication errors. The PTCE® tests familiarity with common terms and the ability to translate them accurately into patient-friendly directions.

Common Sig Code Examples:

- **b.i.d.** – twice daily
- **t.i.d.** – three times daily
- **q.i.d.** – four times daily
- **q6h** – every six hours
- **p.o.** – by mouth
- **PRN** – as needed
- **h.s.** – at bedtime
- **gtt** – drops
- **ad lib.** – as desired

Technicians should avoid error-prone abbreviations and follow institutional "Do Not Use" lists. For example, "U" for units may be mistaken as a zero, leading to tenfold overdoses; always spell out "units." Similarly, trailing zeros (e.g., 1.0 mg) can be misread—use "1 mg" instead.

When transcribing or entering prescriptions electronically, technicians must convert Sig codes into **clear, patient-centered directions** such as "Take one tablet by mouth twice daily." This ensures comprehension and supports patient adherence. Before final verification, every translated instruction should be rechecked against the original prescription for consistency.

Labeling Requirements and Order Verification

Prescription labels serve both legal and clinical purposes, providing patients with essential information and ensuring regulatory compliance. The PTCE® requires understanding of federal labeling standards and the technician's role in maintaining accuracy.

Required Elements on a Prescription Label:

- Pharmacy name, address, and phone number

- Prescription (Rx) number
- Patient's full name
- Prescriber's name
- Medication name, strength, and dosage form
- Directions for use (Sig)
- Date filled or refilled
- Quantity dispensed
- Expiration date or beyond-use date
- Cautionary statements or auxiliary labels

Controlled substance labels must include the federal caution:

"Caution: Federal law prohibits the transfer of this drug to any person other than the patient for whom it was prescribed."

Auxiliary labels communicate safety precautions (e.g., "May cause drowsiness," "Refrigerate," or "Take with food"). Technicians select these based on the medication profile and institutional protocols.

Prior to pharmacist verification, technicians perform a **final product check** by comparing:

1. The prescription label with the original order.
2. The medication stock bottle for correct drug, strength, and dosage form.
3. The filled container's physical contents and label match.

If any mismatch occurs—such as an incorrect NDC number or look-alike product—dispensing must be halted immediately for pharmacist review.

Equipment and Supplies for Drug Administration

Pharmacy technicians must understand the tools and devices used for medication preparation and administration to ensure safe, accurate dispensing. These include both **disposable and reusable** supplies that must be selected and handled based on the medication type, route, and patient needs.

Common Equipment Categories:

- **Measuring devices:** Graduated cylinders, syringes, oral dosing cups, and droppers ensure volume accuracy.
- **Compounding tools:** Mortars, pestles, spatulas, and balances are used for mixing, grinding, and weighing.

- **Administration aids:** Inhaler spacers, oral syringes, insulin syringes, nebulizer kits, and injection filters.
- **Safety equipment:** Gloves, gowns, and masks protect staff during preparation of hazardous substances.

Sterile and nonsterile supplies must be separated and clearly labeled to prevent cross-contamination. Technicians are expected to confirm **calibration** of measuring tools and check for cleanliness or residue before use. When reconstituting powdered medications, sterile diluents must be selected per manufacturer instruction, and all preparation steps recorded in the compounding or dispensing log.

Technicians must also recognize **specialized supplies** for unique patient populations, such as unit-dose packaging for hospitals or safety syringes for immunizations. Familiarity with these devices enhances workflow accuracy and patient safety.

Lot Numbers, Expiration Dates, and Product Integrity

The **lot number** and **expiration date** are key identifiers used to trace medication quality and verify that each product dispensed is within its safe-use period. Every medication container, from manufacturer stock to unit-dose packaging, carries a lot number that links it to a specific production batch. This information is essential for recall response and documentation.

Expiration Date Rules:

- Medications must never be dispensed beyond their printed expiration date.
- For items repackaged in-house, a **beyond-use date (BUD)** must be assigned—typically one year from repackaging or the manufacturer's expiration date, whichever is earlier.
- Refrigerated or reconstituted items often have much shorter BUDs (e.g., 7–14 days).

Technicians are responsible for rotating inventory using the **First Expired, First Out (FEFO)** system and conducting monthly inspections to remove outdated stock. When a medication is recalled, the lot number allows pharmacies to identify and quarantine affected units efficiently.

Visual inspection is also essential. Discoloration, precipitation, or compromised packaging signals possible degradation. Medications that fail visual checks must be segregated and reported to the pharmacist. Maintaining product integrity preserves therapeutic value and aligns with both FDA and DEA requirements for quality assurance.

Chapter 5 – Practice Questions

Questions (1-100)

Q1. Which of the following medications is classified as an angiotensin-converting enzyme (ACE) inhibitor?

A. Amlodipine
B. Lisinopril
C. Losartan
D. Metoprolol

Q2. Which schedule of controlled substances includes drugs with accepted medical use but high potential for abuse, such as oxycodone?

A. Schedule I
B. Schedule II
C. Schedule III
D. Schedule IV

Q3. Which of the following antibiotic classes inhibits bacterial cell wall synthesis?

A. Macrolides
B. Fluoroquinolones
C. Penicillins
D. Tetracyclines

Q4. Which insulin formulation is considered rapid-acting?

A. Insulin glargine
B. Insulin lispro
C. Insulin detemir
D. Insulin NPH

Q5. What is the generic name for the brand drug Plavix®?

A. Clopidogrel
B. Warfarin
C. Apixaban
D. Ticagrelor

Q6. Which of the following medications is a proton-pump inhibitor (PPI)?

A. Ranitidine
B. Omeprazole
C. Famotidine
D. Sucralfate

Q7. Which drug class does furosemide belong to?

A. Thiazide diuretics
B. Loop diuretics
C. Potassium-sparing diuretics
D. Osmotic diuretics

Q8. Metformin primarily lowers blood glucose by which mechanism?

A. Stimulating pancreatic insulin secretion
B. Enhancing insulin sensitivity and reducing hepatic glucose output
C. Inhibiting carbohydrate absorption in intestines
D. Mimicking GLP-1 activity

Q9. What is the therapeutic classification of albuterol?

A. Antihistamine
B. Beta-2 agonist

C. Corticosteroid
D. Leukotriene inhibitor

Q10. Which drug is most associated with a dry, persistent cough as a side effect?
A. Losartan
B. Hydrochlorothiazide
C. Amlodipine
D. Lisinopril

Q11. Which of the following medications is a selective serotonin reuptake inhibitor (SSRI)?
A. Venlafaxine
B. Fluoxetine
C. Amitriptyline
D. Bupropion

Q12. Which vitamin deficiency is most associated with prolonged isoniazid therapy?
A. Vitamin B1 (thiamine)
B. Vitamin B6 (pyridoxine)
C. Vitamin B12 (cobalamin)
D. Vitamin K

Q13. Which drug is contraindicated in patients with a sulfa allergy?
A. Furosemide
B. Amoxicillin
C. Cephalexin
D. Azithromycin

Q14. Which of the following opioid analgesics is available as a transdermal patch?
A. Hydrocodone
B. Oxycodone
C. Fentanyl
D. Codeine

Q15. Which of the following drugs is classified as a benzodiazepine?
A. Zolpidem
B. Lorazepam
C. Buspirone
D. Trazodone

Q16. Which medication requires INR monitoring due to its narrow therapeutic index?
A. Clopidogrel
B. Warfarin
C. Apixaban
D. Dabigatran

Q17. Which medication is commonly used as an HMG-CoA reductase inhibitor?
A. Gemfibrozil
B. Atorvastatin
C. Ezetimibe
D. Niacin

Q18. Which corticosteroid is commonly prescribed for asthma maintenance via inhalation?
A. Prednisone
B. Hydrocortisone
C. Fluticasone
D. Dexamethasone

Q19. Which class of drug is used to treat hyperthyroidism?

A. Thyroid hormone replacement
B. Beta-blockers
C. Antithyroid agents like methimazole
D. Corticosteroids

Q20. What is the mechanism of action of amlodipine?
A. Beta-blockade
B. Calcium-channel blockade in vascular smooth muscle
C. ACE inhibition
D. Alpha-adrenergic antagonism

Q21. Which of the following medications is classified as an anticoagulant that directly inhibits Factor Xa?
A. Warfarin
B. Dabigatran
C. Apixaban
D. Heparin

Q22. Which medication is used to treat hypothyroidism?
A. Methimazole
B. Propylthiouracil
C. Levothyroxine
D. Prednisolone

Q23. What is the brand name for montelukast?
A. Singulair®
B. Symbicort®
C. Spiriva®
D. Serevent®

Q24. Which antiepileptic drug is known to cause gingival hyperplasia as a side effect?
A. Levetiracetam
B. Phenytoin
C. Valproic acid
D. Topiramate

Q25. Which medication is used as an antidote for acetaminophen overdose?
A. Flumazenil
B. Naloxone
C. N-acetylcysteine
D. Atropine

Q26. Which of the following medications is an alpha-1 blocker used for benign prostatic hyperplasia (BPH)?
A. Finasteride
B. Tamsulosin
C. Oxybutynin
D. Tolterodine

Q27. Which antidepressant also aids in smoking cessation therapy?
A. Sertraline
B. Bupropion
C. Amitriptyline
D. Escitalopram

Q28. Which medication should be avoided in patients with a true penicillin allergy?
A. Cephalexin

B. Azithromycin
C. Ciprofloxacin
D. Doxycycline

Q29. Which of the following drugs is an antipsychotic with a high risk of agranulocytosis?
A. Risperidone
B. Clozapine
C. Quetiapine
D. Olanzapine

Q30. Which of these medications is used to treat type 1 diabetes mellitus?
A. Glipizide
B. Metformin
C. Sitagliptin
D. Insulin glargine

Q31. Which of the following antibiotics belongs to the macrolide class?
A. Doxycycline
B. Azithromycin
C. Amoxicillin
D. Levofloxacin

Q32. What is the mechanism of action of proton pump inhibitors?
A. Blocking histamine H_2 receptors
B. Neutralizing stomach acid directly
C. Inhibiting gastric proton pump H^+/K^+-ATPase
D. Stimulating gastric mucosal secretion

Q33. Which drug is used to prevent chemotherapy-induced nausea and vomiting?
A. Ondansetron
B. Loperamide
C. Promethazine
D. Diphenhydramine

Q34. Which of these drugs is a corticosteroid that can be administered orally for inflammation?
A. Methylprednisolone
B. Fluticasone
C. Hydrocortisone cream
D. Budesonide inhaler

Q35. Which diuretic conserves potassium during its action?
A. Furosemide
B. Hydrochlorothiazide
C. Spironolactone
D. Bumetanide

Q36. Which of the following drugs is used to treat gout by lowering uric acid production?
A. Colchicine
B. Allopurinol
C. Probenecid
D. Naproxen

Q37. Which medication is a calcium channel blocker used for arrhythmia management?
A. Verapamil
B. Metoprolol
C. Lisinopril
D. Diltiazem

Q38. Which antibiotic is associated with photosensitivity reactions?
A. Ciprofloxacin
B. Amoxicillin
C. Azithromycin
D. Clindamycin
Q39. What is the mechanism of action for digoxin?
A. Beta-adrenergic blockade
B. Calcium-channel inhibition
C. Sodium-potassium ATPase inhibition increasing contractility
D. ACE inhibition
Q40. Which class of antidepressants carries the highest risk for anticholinergic side effects?
A. SSRIs
B. SNRIs
C. MAOIs
D. Tricyclic antidepressants
Q41. Which of the following medications is a potassium supplement?
A. Klor-Con®
B. Lasix®
C. Microzide®
D. Aldactone®
Q42. Which antibiotic class can cause tendon rupture, particularly in older adults?
A. Penicillins
B. Fluoroquinolones
C. Macrolides
D. Cephalosporins
Q43. Which of these medications is used to treat bipolar disorder and requires serum level monitoring?
A. Sertraline
B. Lithium
C. Aripiprazole
D. Lamotrigine
Q44. Which of the following medications is a selective beta-1 blocker?
A. Propranolol
B. Carvedilol
C. Metoprolol
D. Labetalol
Q45. Which of these drugs is classified as an anticonvulsant and mood stabilizer?
A. Gabapentin
B. Valproic acid
C. Diazepam
D. Sertraline
Q46. Which medication should be avoided with grapefruit juice due to CYP3A4 inhibition?
A. Atenolol
B. Simvastatin
C. Hydrochlorothiazide
D. Lisinopril
Q47. Which medication is classified as an opioid antagonist?
A. Methadone

B. Naloxone
C. Fentanyl
D. Buprenorphine

Q48. What is the brand name for the generic drug sertraline?
A. Prozac®
B. Zoloft®
C. Lexapro®
D. Celexa®

Q49. Which medication is classified as an antifungal agent?
A. Metronidazole
B. Acyclovir
C. Fluconazole
D. Oseltamivir

Q50. Which medication is a nonsteroidal anti-inflammatory drug (NSAID)?
A. Acetaminophen
B. Ibuprofen
C. Hydrocodone
D. Tramadol

Q51. Which of the following medications is used as a bronchodilator in COPD?
A. Tiotropium
B. Loratadine
C. Cetirizine
D. Diphenhydramine

Q52. Which drug is a serotonin-norepinephrine reuptake inhibitor (SNRI)?
A. Escitalopram
B. Venlafaxine
C. Trazodone
D. Mirtazapine

Q53. Which of the following medications is commonly used to treat opioid dependence?
A. Methadone
B. Fentanyl
C. Diazepam
D. Midazolam

Q54. Which of these medications treats hypertension by blocking angiotensin II receptors?
A. Amlodipine
B. Lisinopril
C. Losartan
D. Metoprolol

Q55. Which drug is used to prevent motion sickness?
A. Lorazepam
B. Scopolamine
C. Fexofenadine
D. Montelukast

Q56. Which of the following is a muscle relaxant?
A. Baclofen
B. Celecoxib
C. Sertraline
D. Prednisone

Q57. Which medication is used for emergency treatment of severe hypoglycemia?
A. Insulin lispro
B. Glucagon
C. Metformin
D. Pioglitazone
Q58. Which of the following is an over-the-counter H_2 receptor antagonist?
A. Omeprazole
B. Famotidine
C. Lansoprazole
D. Esomeprazole
Q59. Which of the following medications is a selective serotonin and norepinephrine reuptake inhibitor (SNRI)?
A. Fluoxetine
B. Sertraline
C. Venlafaxine
D. Trazodone
Q60. Which of these medications is an oral contraceptive containing estrogen and progestin?
A. Medroxyprogesterone
B. Drospirenone/ethinyl estradiol
C. Levonorgestrel
D. Clomiphene
Q61. Which of the following antipsychotic medications has the lowest risk of extrapyramidal symptoms?
A. Haloperidol
B. Risperidone
C. Clozapine
D. Fluphenazine
Q62. Which of these medications is used to treat hypertension and benign prostatic hyperplasia (BPH)?
A. Lisinopril
B. Doxazosin
C. Amlodipine
D. Metoprolol
Q63. Which medication is an anticonvulsant also indicated for neuropathic pain?
A. Carbamazepine
B. Gabapentin
C. Valproic acid
D. Ethosuximide
Q64. Which medication is used for migraine prophylaxis and hypertension?
A. Sumatriptan
B. Propranolol
C. Rizatriptan
D. Topiramate
Q65. Which drug is used to treat urinary tract infections and may cause urine discoloration?
A. Ciprofloxacin
B. Nitrofurantoin
C. Trimethoprim
D. Amoxicillin

Q66. Which of the following is a benzodiazepine used for seizure emergencies?
A. Lorazepam
B. Trazodone
C. Buspirone
D. Hydroxyzine
Q67. Which medication is used to treat hyperlipidemia by inhibiting cholesterol absorption in the intestine?
A. Ezetimibe
B. Atorvastatin
C. Gemfibrozil
D. Niacin
Q68. Which of these drugs is classified as an angiotensin receptor blocker (ARB)?
A. Lisinopril
B. Losartan
C. Amlodipine
D. Atenolol
Q69. Which antibiotic is known for causing "Red Man Syndrome" if infused too quickly?
A. Vancomycin
B. Gentamicin
C. Ceftriaxone
D. Azithromycin
Q70. Which of these medications is classified as a proton pump inhibitor?
A. Ranitidine
B. Lansoprazole
C. Cimetidine
D. Misoprostol
Q71. Which medication is used as an antitussive agent?
A. Dextromethorphan
B. Guaifenesin
C. Pseudoephedrine
D. Loratadine
Q72. Which antibiotic requires counseling to avoid alcohol during therapy?
A. Metronidazole
B. Doxycycline
C. Azithromycin
D. Cephalexin
Q73. Which medication is classified as an atypical antipsychotic?
A. Haloperidol
B. Chlorpromazine
C. Quetiapine
D. Fluphenazine
Q74. Which of these medications is a short-acting beta-2 agonist?
A. Salmeterol
B. Albuterol
C. Formoterol
D. Tiotropium
Q75. Which of the following drugs is a thyroid hormone used in hypothyroidism?
A. Methimazole

B. Propylthiouracil
C. Levothyroxine
D. Prednisone

Q76. Which antidepressant carries a risk of serotonin syndrome when combined with MAOIs?

A. Fluoxetine
B. Bupropion
C. Trazodone
D. Mirtazapine

Q77. Which drug is classified as an anticoagulant that enhances antithrombin activity?

A. Heparin
B. Warfarin
C. Apixaban
D. Dabigatran

Q78. Which antibiotic should not be taken with dairy products due to chelation?

A. Azithromycin
B. Tetracycline
C. Metronidazole
D. Clindamycin

Q79. Which of the following medications is used to reduce uric acid levels in gout prevention?

A. Colchicine
B. Allopurinol
C. Naproxen
D. Prednisone

Q80. Which of these medications is a nasal corticosteroid for allergic rhinitis?

A. Fluticasone
B. Loratadine
C. Pseudoephedrine
D. Montelukast

Q81. Which class of medications does amoxicillin belong to?

A. Macrolides
B. Penicillins
C. Fluoroquinolones
D. Tetracyclines

Q82. Which of the following drugs is used to treat opioid-induced constipation?

A. Docusate sodium
B. Naloxegol
C. Senna
D. Lactulose

Q83. Which antidiabetic drug belongs to the sulfonylurea class?

A. Metformin
B. Glipizide
C. Sitagliptin
D. Pioglitazone

Q84. Which of these drugs is a dopamine precursor used in Parkinson's disease?

A. Benztropine
B. Carbidopa/Levodopa
C. Ropinirole
D. Selegiline

Q85. Which medication is commonly prescribed for neuropathic pain associated with diabetes?
A. Duloxetine
B. Lorazepam
C. Paroxetine
D. Clonazepam
Q86. Which of the following is a long-acting insulin?
A. Insulin aspart
B. Insulin lispro
C. Insulin glargine
D. Insulin regular
Q87. Which class of medications is used to lower triglycerides?
A. Fibrates
B. Statins
C. ACE inhibitors
D. ARBs
Q88. Which of these medications is used to prevent peptic ulcers in patients on NSAIDs?
A. Sucralfate
B. Misoprostol
C. Omeprazole
D. Ranitidine
Q89. Which of the following drugs is classified as a serotonin antagonist and reuptake inhibitor (SARI)?
A. Trazodone
B. Sertraline
C. Venlafaxine
D. Bupropion
Q90. Which of these antibiotics is classified as a cephalosporin?
A. Doxycycline
B. Cephalexin
C. Levofloxacin
D. Erythromycin
Q91. Which drug is a selective alpha-2 adrenergic agonist used for hypertension?
A. Clonidine
B. Doxazosin
C. Labetalol
D. Propranolol
Q92. Which of these medications is an anticoagulant that inhibits vitamin K–dependent clotting factors?
A. Warfarin
B. Heparin
C. Apixaban
D. Rivaroxaban
Q93. Which of these medications is an ACE inhibitor?
A. Losartan
B. Lisinopril
C. Amlodipine
D. Metoprolol
Q94. Which medication is commonly used to treat anxiety disorders and is non-sedating?
A. Alprazolam

B. Buspirone
C. Lorazepam
D. Diazepam

Q95. Which of the following medications is used to lower uric acid levels?

A. Colchicine
B. Allopurinol
C. Naproxen
D. Prednisone

Q96. Which drug is a leukotriene receptor antagonist?

A. Albuterol
B. Montelukast
C. Fluticasone
D. Tiotropium

Q97. Which of the following medications is used for ADHD and acts as a stimulant?

A. Atomoxetine
B. Methylphenidate
C. Clonidine
D. Bupropion

Q98. Which medication is classified as a non-opioid analgesic with antipyretic activity?

A. Ibuprofen
B. Acetaminophen
C. Tramadol
D. Naproxen

Q99. Which of the following medications is an antiplatelet agent?

A. Clopidogrel
B. Warfarin
C. Heparin
D. Apixaban

Q100. Which drug is used as an antidote for benzodiazepine overdose?

A. Naloxone
B. Flumazenil
C. Atropine
D. Acetylcysteine

Answer key and Explanation (1-100)

Q1. Answer: B

Explanation: Lisinopril is an ACE inhibitor that lowers blood pressure by blocking angiotensin I conversion. Losartan is an ARB, amlodipine a calcium-channel blocker, and metoprolol a beta-blocker. ACE inhibitors also protect kidneys in diabetic nephropathy, differentiating them from other antihypertensive classes through their unique renal-protective mechanism.

Q2. Answer: B

Explanation: Schedule II drugs have recognized medical use yet carry a high risk for abuse and dependence. Oxycodone and morphine are examples. Schedule I drugs lack accepted medical use, while Schedule III and IV contain substances with decreasing abuse potential, demonstrating the tiered control framework established under the Controlled Substances Act.

Q3. Answer: C

Explanation: Penicillins act by inhibiting bacterial cell-wall synthesis, causing cell lysis and death. Macrolides inhibit protein synthesis, fluoroquinolones block DNA gyrase, and tetracyclines prevent ribosomal tRNA binding. Understanding mechanisms aids in preventing duplicate therapy and managing resistance when multiple antibiotics are prescribed simultaneously.

Q4. Answer: B

Explanation: Insulin lispro is rapid-acting, typically onset within 15 minutes and duration 3–5 hours, ideal for pre-meal glucose control. Glargine and detemir are long-acting, providing basal coverage, while NPH is intermediate. Correct identification supports patient counseling on timing to prevent hypoglycemia associated with improper meal synchronization.

Q5. Answer: A

Explanation: Plavix® contains clopidogrel, an antiplatelet agent that inhibits ADP-mediated platelet aggregation. Warfarin and apixaban are anticoagulants targeting clotting factors, while ticagrelor acts similarly to clopidogrel but with reversible binding. Technicians must recognize this distinction when substituting or identifying look-alike antithrombotic medications.

Q6. Answer: B

Explanation: Omeprazole, a PPI, irreversibly inhibits the H^+/K^+ ATPase in gastric parietal cells, suppressing acid production longer than H_2 antagonists like ranitidine or famotidine. Sucralfate forms a protective barrier but does not reduce acid secretion. Recognizing PPIs is crucial for managing GERD and ulcer therapy scheduling.

Q7. Answer: B

Explanation: Furosemide is a loop diuretic acting in the ascending loop of Henle to inhibit $Na^+/K^+/2Cl^-$ reabsorption, producing potent diuresis. Thiazides work distally, potassium-sparing diuretics conserve K^+, and osmotic agents like mannitol increase filtrate osmolarity. Loop diuretics are preferred in acute pulmonary edema and require electrolyte monitoring.

Q8. Answer: B

Explanation: Metformin, a biguanide, decreases hepatic gluconeogenesis and improves peripheral insulin sensitivity without increasing insulin release. Sulfonylureas stimulate pancreatic secretion, acarbose inhibits carbohydrate absorption, and GLP-1 agonists enhance incretin action. Understanding mechanisms reduces duplicate therapy risk and guides monitoring for lactic acidosis in renal impairment.

Q9. Answer: B

Explanation: Albuterol is a short-acting β_2-adrenergic agonist that relaxes bronchial smooth muscle for rapid relief of asthma symptoms. Corticosteroids provide anti-inflammatory control, while leukotriene inhibitors prevent mediator release. Technicians must distinguish rescue from maintenance agents to ensure proper labeling and patient counseling on inhaler use.

Q10. Answer: D

Explanation: Lisinopril, an ACE inhibitor, increases bradykinin levels leading to a dry cough. Losartan, an ARB, does not produce this effect and is often substituted when the symptom occurs. Amlodipine and hydrochlorothiazide rarely cause cough, highlighting mechanistic differences between ACE and ARB antihypertensive agents.

Q11. Answer: B

Explanation: Fluoxetine is an SSRI used for depression and anxiety, inhibiting serotonin reuptake in CNS synapses. Venlafaxine is an SNRI, amitriptyline a tricyclic, and bupropion a dopamine-norepinephrine reuptake inhibitor. Recognizing these differences prevents therapeutic duplication and serotonin syndrome when multiple antidepressants are prescribed.

Q12. Answer: B

Explanation: Isoniazid impairs pyridoxine metabolism, causing neuropathy preventable with vitamin B6 supplementation. Other vitamins serve different roles—thiamine in carbohydrate metabolism, B12 in hematopoiesis, and K in coagulation. Technicians should flag isoniazid prescriptions for supplement verification to avoid preventable adverse effects during TB therapy.

Q13. Answer: A

Explanation: Furosemide contains a sulfonamide moiety, posing risk for cross-reactivity in sulfa-allergic patients. Amoxicillin and cephalexin are β-lactams, while azithromycin is a macrolide, none sharing that structure. Verification of allergies before dispensing loop or thiazide diuretics is critical for preventing hypersensitivity reactions.

Q14. Answer: C

Explanation: Fentanyl is available in transdermal form for chronic pain management, offering steady systemic delivery. Hydrocodone and oxycodone are oral formulations, and codeine is used in combination analgesics or cough suppressants. Proper handling and disposal of patches are vital to prevent accidental exposure and overdose.

Q15. Answer: B

Explanation: Lorazepam is a benzodiazepine that enhances GABA activity to produce anxiolytic and sedative effects. Zolpidem is a non-benzodiazepine hypnotic, buspirone a serotonin agonist, and trazodone a serotonin antagonist used for sleep. Technicians must store benzodiazepines securely and monitor refills as controlled substances (Schedule IV).

Q16. Answer: B

Explanation: Warfarin inhibits vitamin K-dependent clotting factors and requires INR testing to maintain efficacy and avoid bleeding. Clopidogrel and apixaban do not require routine INR monitoring. Technicians should ensure consistency in warfarin brand and diet counseling due to interactions with vitamin K-rich foods and numerous drugs.

Q17. Answer: B

Explanation: Atorvastatin lowers LDL by inhibiting HMG-CoA reductase, reducing cholesterol biosynthesis. Gemfibrozil targets triglycerides, ezetimibe blocks intestinal absorption, and niacin reduces VLDL production. Monitoring for muscle pain and LFT changes is essential to identify rare myopathy and hepatotoxicity associated with statins.

Q18. Answer: C

Explanation: Fluticasone is an inhaled corticosteroid providing localized anti-inflammatory action for asthma maintenance. Prednisone and dexamethasone are systemic steroids, while hydrocortisone is topical or IV. Inhaled steroids reduce exacerbations with fewer systemic effects but require rinse-and-spit counseling to prevent oral candidiasis.

Q19. Answer: C

Explanation: Methimazole inhibits thyroid hormone synthesis, making it the first-line therapy for hyperthyroidism. Beta-blockers control symptoms only, whereas levothyroxine is for hypothyroidism.

Technicians must remind patients about consistent dosing and monitoring for signs of agranulocytosis such as fever or sore throat.

Q20. Answer: B

Explanation: Amlodipine blocks calcium entry into vascular smooth muscle, leading to vasodilation and reduced blood pressure. Unlike beta-blockers, it does not affect heart rate significantly. ACE inhibitors reduce angiotensin II production instead. Knowledge of mechanism guides identification of additive hypotensive effects in polypharmacy.

Q21. Answer: C

Explanation: Apixaban inhibits Factor Xa, preventing thrombin formation and clot development. Unlike warfarin, it doesn't require INR monitoring. Dabigatran inhibits thrombin directly, and heparin acts indirectly through antithrombin. Technicians must check renal function and counsel on adherence, as missed doses rapidly reduce anticoagulant protection.

Q22. Answer: C

Explanation: Levothyroxine is a synthetic form of T_4 used to replace deficient thyroid hormone in hypothyroidism. Methimazole and propylthiouracil treat hyperthyroidism by inhibiting hormone synthesis. Prednisolone is a corticosteroid unrelated to thyroid regulation. Consistent daily timing before breakfast ensures stable absorption and optimal hormone balance.

Q23. Answer: A

Explanation: Montelukast, marketed as Singulair®, is a leukotriene receptor antagonist used for asthma maintenance and allergic rhinitis. Symbicort® combines a corticosteroid with a long-acting beta agonist, while Spiriva® and Serevent® act as bronchodilators. Recognizing brand–generic pairs helps prevent substitution errors in asthma control regimens.

Q24. Answer: B

Explanation: Phenytoin commonly causes gingival hyperplasia, requiring patients to maintain good oral hygiene. Valproic acid may cause hepatotoxicity, topiramate induces weight loss, and levetiracetam is well tolerated neurologically. Recognizing adverse effect profiles helps technicians reinforce adherence and monitor for preventable dental complications.

Q25. Answer: C

Explanation: N-acetylcysteine replenishes hepatic glutathione, neutralizing acetaminophen's toxic metabolite and preventing liver damage. Flumazenil reverses benzodiazepines, naloxone counteracts opioids, and atropine treats organophosphate poisoning. Technicians should recognize its emergency role and ensure timely compounding or preparation in hospital settings.

Q26. Answer: B

Explanation: Tamsulosin relaxes smooth muscle in the prostate and bladder neck, improving urinary flow in BPH. Finasteride reduces prostate size hormonally, while oxybutynin and tolterodine treat overactive bladder. Technicians should warn patients about orthostatic hypotension risk when initiating alpha-blocker therapy.

Q27. Answer: B

Explanation: Bupropion inhibits norepinephrine and dopamine reuptake, reducing nicotine cravings and withdrawal symptoms. SSRIs like sertraline and escitalopram treat mood disorders but not nicotine addiction. Amitriptyline, a tricyclic, has sedative effects unsuitable for cessation. Pharmacists monitor for seizure risk, particularly in predisposed patients.

Q28. Answer: A

Explanation: Cephalexin, a first-generation cephalosporin, may cause cross-reactivity in patients with penicillin allergy. Azithromycin, ciprofloxacin, and doxycycline belong to different antibiotic classes. Although modern data suggest low cross-reactivity, verification of allergy severity remains a critical technician safety step before dispensing.

Q29. Answer: B

Explanation: Clozapine carries a black box warning for agranulocytosis, necessitating routine CBC monitoring. Risperidone, quetiapine, and olanzapine have metabolic but not hematologic risks. Technicians should ensure REMS program compliance and patient education about infection symptoms requiring urgent evaluation.

Q30. Answer: D

Explanation: Insulin glargine provides long-acting basal insulin essential for type 1 diabetes management, as endogenous insulin is absent. Glipizide, metformin, and sitagliptin rely on pancreatic or metabolic function present in type 2 diabetes. Proper injection technique and site rotation prevent lipohypertrophy.

Q31. Answer: B

Explanation: Azithromycin, a macrolide, inhibits bacterial protein synthesis by binding the 50S ribosomal subunit. Doxycycline is a tetracycline, amoxicillin a beta-lactam, and levofloxacin a fluoroquinolone. Macrolides are often used for respiratory infections and safe in penicillin-allergic patients, though they can prolong QT intervals.

Q32. Answer: C

Explanation: PPIs irreversibly inhibit H^+/K^+-ATPase in gastric parietal cells, suppressing acid secretion. H_2 blockers like famotidine only block histamine-mediated release, while antacids neutralize acid directly. PPIs provide superior healing in GERD and ulcers, requiring consistent dosing 30–60 minutes before meals.

Q33. Answer: A

Explanation: Ondansetron, a 5-HT_3 receptor antagonist, prevents serotonin-mediated nausea common in chemotherapy. Promethazine and diphenhydramine are antihistamines with sedative properties, while loperamide treats diarrhea. Technicians prepare ondansetron in both oral and IV forms, verifying dose timing with chemotherapy sessions for effectiveness.

Q34. Answer: A

Explanation: Methylprednisolone is available orally and parenterally for systemic inflammation. Fluticasone and budesonide are inhaled, targeting respiratory inflammation locally locally, while hydrocortisone cream is topical. Systemic steroids require tapering and monitoring for adrenal suppression, emphasizing technician attention to therapy duration instructions.

Q35. Answer: C

Explanation: Spironolactone is a potassium-sparing diuretic that antagonizes aldosterone at the distal nephron, conserving potassium. Loop and thiazide diuretics cause potassium loss. Monitoring for hyperkalemia is essential, especially when combined with ACE inhibitors or potassium supplements. Counsel patients to avoid excess dietary potassium intake.

Q36. Answer: B

Explanation: Allopurinol inhibits xanthine oxidase, reducing uric acid formation and preventing gout flares. Colchicine treats acute attacks, probenecid increases uric acid excretion, and naproxen is anti-inflammatory only. Technicians should ensure hydration counseling and note dose adjustments in renal impairment.

Q37. Answer: D

Explanation: Diltiazem, a non-dihydropyridine calcium channel blocker, slows AV conduction and reduces heart rate. Verapamil shares similar action but stronger cardiac suppression, while metoprolol is a beta-blocker and lisinopril an ACE inhibitor. Accurate selection ensures appropriate therapy for rate control in atrial fibrillation.

Q38. Answer: A

Explanation: Ciprofloxacin, a fluoroquinolone, increases photosensitivity risk, necessitating sunscreen counseling. Tetracyclines share this risk, but amoxicillin, azithromycin, and clindamycin generally do not.

Technicians should remind patients to avoid tanning beds and prolonged sun exposure during therapy to prevent phototoxic skin reactions.

Q39. Answer: C

Explanation: Digoxin inhibits the Na^+/K^+ ATPase, increasing intracellular calcium and improving cardiac contractility. It also slows AV nodal conduction, useful in heart failure and atrial fibrillation. Monitoring for toxicity and maintaining consistent brand substitution are vital due to its narrow therapeutic window.

Q40. Answer: D

Explanation: Tricyclic antidepressants (TCAs) such as amitriptyline cause pronounced anticholinergic effects—dry mouth, constipation, blurred vision, urinary retention—due to muscarinic blockade. SSRIs and SNRIs are better tolerated, while MAOIs pose dietary interaction risks. Recognizing these profiles helps technicians flag potential adverse effects in elderly patients.

Q41. Answer: A

Explanation: Klor-Con® contains potassium chloride, used to prevent or treat hypokalemia, especially in patients on loop or thiazide diuretics. Lasix® (furosemide) and Microzide® (hydrochlorothiazide) cause potassium loss, while Aldactone® (spironolactone) conserves potassium. Technicians should ensure proper dosing and advise patients not to crush extended-release tablets.

Q42. Answer: B

Explanation: Fluoroquinolones such as ciprofloxacin and levofloxacin may cause tendon inflammation or rupture, especially in the Achilles tendon. Penicillins, macrolides, and cephalosporins do not share this risk. Technicians should counsel patients to report sudden tendon pain and avoid strenuous activity during therapy.

Q43. Answer: B

Explanation: Lithium stabilizes mood by affecting neurotransmitter balance but has a narrow therapeutic index, requiring regular serum level and renal monitoring. Sertraline treats depression, aripiprazole is an atypical antipsychotic, and lamotrigine is an anticonvulsant mood stabilizer without strict serum monitoring requirements.

Q44. Answer: C

Explanation: Metoprolol selectively blocks beta-1 receptors in the heart, reducing heart rate and contractility. Propranolol and carvedilol block both beta-1 and beta-2 receptors, while labetalol adds alpha-blocking properties. Beta-1 selectivity minimizes bronchoconstriction risk, making metoprolol safer for asthmatic patients.

Q45. Answer: B

Explanation: Valproic acid treats seizure disorders and bipolar disorder by increasing GABA levels in the brain. Gabapentin is for neuropathic pain, diazepam is a benzodiazepine, and sertraline is an SSRI antidepressant. Monitoring liver enzymes and platelet counts is essential due to valproic acid's hepatotoxic risk.

Q46. Answer: B

Explanation: Simvastatin's metabolism is inhibited by grapefruit juice, raising plasma concentrations and myopathy risk. Atenolol, hydrochlorothiazide, and lisinopril are unaffected. Technicians should warn patients to avoid grapefruit products with most statins and calcium channel blockers to prevent serious drug-food interactions.

Q47. Answer: B

Explanation: Naloxone rapidly reverses opioid overdose by competitively blocking opioid receptors. Methadone and buprenorphine are partial agonists used for dependence treatment, and fentanyl is a full agonist. Technicians dispensing naloxone must instruct on nasal spray or injection use in emergency overdose scenarios.

Q48. Answer: B

Explanation: Sertraline is marketed as Zoloft®, an SSRI for depression, OCD, and anxiety. Prozac® is fluoxetine, Lexapro® is escitalopram, and Celexa® is citalopram. Recognizing common brand-generic pairs is critical for technicians to ensure accurate dispensing and patient counseling on therapy adherence.

Q49. Answer: C

Explanation: Fluconazole inhibits fungal cytochrome P450 enzymes, disrupting cell membrane synthesis. Metronidazole targets anaerobic bacteria, acyclovir treats herpes viruses, and oseltamivir is antiviral for influenza. Technicians must confirm antifungal dosage adjustments for renal impairment and counsel patients on potential hepatotoxicity.

Q50. Answer: B

Explanation: Ibuprofen inhibits cyclooxygenase (COX) enzymes, reducing prostaglandin synthesis responsible for inflammation and pain. Acetaminophen lacks anti-inflammatory properties, while hydrocodone and tramadol act as opioids. Patients should avoid concurrent NSAIDs to reduce GI bleeding and nephrotoxicity risks from cumulative COX inhibition.

Q51. Answer: A

Explanation: Tiotropium is a long-acting anticholinergic bronchodilator (LAMA) that relaxes airway muscles, improving airflow in COPD. Loratadine and cetirizine are antihistamines for allergies, and diphenhydramine is a sedating antihistamine. Proper inhaler use and daily adherence maximize tiotropium's bronchodilation benefits.

Q52. Answer: B

Explanation: Venlafaxine blocks reuptake of both serotonin and norepinephrine, enhancing neurotransmission. Escitalopram is an SSRI, trazodone is a serotonin antagonist and reuptake inhibitor, and mirtazapine is a presynaptic alpha-2 blocker. SNRIs require gradual tapering to avoid withdrawal symptoms and blood pressure monitoring.

Q53. Answer: A

Explanation: Methadone, a long-acting opioid agonist, prevents withdrawal symptoms and reduces cravings in opioid use disorder. Fentanyl is a potent analgesic, while diazepam and midazolam are benzodiazepines. Methadone must be dispensed in certified programs under strict DEA regulations.

Q54. Answer: C

Explanation: Losartan blocks angiotensin II receptors, preventing vasoconstriction and aldosterone release, lowering blood pressure. Lisinopril inhibits ACE, amlodipine blocks calcium channels, and metoprolol slows heart rate. ARBs are useful when ACE inhibitors cause cough or angioedema, offering comparable cardiovascular protection.

Q55. Answer: B

Explanation: Scopolamine, an anticholinergic patch, blocks acetylcholine at vestibular receptors, preventing nausea and dizziness from motion. Lorazepam is anxiolytic, fexofenadine treats allergies, and montelukast is an asthma medication. Technicians advise application 4 hours before travel and handwashing after handling patches.

Q56. Answer: A

Explanation: Baclofen reduces spasticity by activating GABA-B receptors in the spinal cord, decreasing muscle reflexes. Celecoxib is an NSAID, sertraline an antidepressant, and prednisone a corticosteroid. Abrupt withdrawal may cause rebound spasticity, so dose tapering under supervision is critical.

Q57. Answer: B

Explanation: Glucagon promotes hepatic glycogen breakdown, rapidly increasing blood glucose in unconscious or unresponsive hypoglycemic patients. Insulin lowers glucose, while metformin and pioglitazone manage chronic hyperglycemia. Technicians should educate caregivers on proper injection preparation and immediate post-recovery nutrition.

Q58. Answer: B

Explanation: Famotidine is an OTC H_2 blocker that reduces stomach acid for heartburn and GERD. Omeprazole, lansoprazole, and esomeprazole are PPIs requiring scheduled dosing. Technicians should caution against long-term unsupervised use and recommend physician consultation for persistent symptoms.

Q59. Answer: C

Explanation: Venlafaxine increases both serotonin and norepinephrine levels to treat depression and anxiety disorders. Fluoxetine and sertraline are SSRIs, while trazodone mainly blocks serotonin receptors. Blood pressure monitoring is important as venlafaxine can increase BP at higher doses.

Q60. Answer: B

Explanation: Drospirenone/ethinyl estradiol combines synthetic estrogen and progestin to inhibit ovulation and regulate cycles. Medroxyprogesterone is injectable, levonorgestrel is emergency contraception, and clomiphene induces ovulation. Missed doses increase pregnancy risk, requiring adherence counseling.

Q61. Answer: C

Explanation: Clozapine, an atypical antipsychotic, causes minimal extrapyramidal side effects due to low dopamine receptor affinity. Haloperidol and fluphenazine are typical agents with high EPS risk, while risperidone carries moderate risk. Technicians must ensure regular blood count monitoring due to clozapine's agranulocytosis potential.

Q62. Answer: B

Explanation: Doxazosin is an alpha-1 adrenergic blocker that reduces vascular resistance and relaxes prostatic smooth muscle. Lisinopril and amlodipine lower blood pressure but do not affect urinary symptoms. Monitoring for first-dose hypotension is vital, particularly in patients initiating alpha-blocker therapy.

Q63. Answer: B

Explanation: Gabapentin modulates calcium channels, reducing neuronal excitability in both seizures and neuropathic pain. Carbamazepine also treats pain but has more interactions; valproic acid is primarily for generalized seizures. Gabapentin requires renal dose adjustment and caution regarding sedation or dizziness.

Q64. Answer: B

Explanation: Propranolol, a non-selective beta-blocker, prevents migraines by stabilizing vascular tone and reduces blood pressure. Sumatriptan and rizatriptan are abortive agents for acute attacks, while topiramate is also preventive but classified as an anticonvulsant. Monitoring heart rate and fatigue is recommended.

Q65. Answer: B

Explanation: Nitrofurantoin treats lower urinary tract infections and can cause harmless brownish urine discoloration. Ciprofloxacin and trimethoprim serve as alternatives, while amoxicillin is less effective against resistant strains. Patients should take nitrofurantoin with food to enhance absorption and reduce gastrointestinal upset.

Q66. Answer: A

Explanation: Lorazepam acts rapidly by enhancing GABA activity, making it effective for status epilepticus and acute anxiety. Trazodone is an antidepressant, buspirone treats generalized anxiety without sedation, and hydroxyzine is an antihistamine. Technicians ensure controlled substance storage and correct labeling for IV or oral formulations.

Q67. Answer: A

Explanation: Ezetimibe blocks intestinal absorption of cholesterol, complementing statin therapy. Atorvastatin inhibits hepatic synthesis, gemfibrozil lowers triglycerides, and niacin reduces VLDL production. Combining ezetimibe with statins improves LDL reduction but requires liver function monitoring for additive hepatotoxic risk.

Q68. Answer: B
Explanation: Losartan blocks angiotensin II receptors, reducing vasoconstriction and aldosterone release. Lisinopril inhibits ACE, amlodipine is a calcium-channel blocker, and atenolol is a beta-blocker. ARBs are alternatives when ACE inhibitors cause cough or angioedema, offering similar antihypertensive efficacy and renal protection.
Q69. Answer: A
Explanation: Vancomycin can cause histamine-mediated flushing called Red Man Syndrome during rapid IV infusion. Slowing the rate and premedicating with antihistamines prevents this reaction. Gentamicin risks nephrotoxicity, ceftriaxone is a cephalosporin, and azithromycin is a macrolide without this effect.
Q70. Answer: B
Explanation: Lansoprazole suppresses gastric acid secretion by inhibiting the H^+/K^+ ATPase enzyme in the stomach lining. Ranitidine and cimetidine are H_2 blockers, while misoprostol is a prostaglandin analog used for ulcer prevention. PPIs offer longer relief but may reduce calcium absorption long-term.
Q71. Answer: A
Explanation: Dextromethorphan suppresses the cough reflex by acting on the medulla, unlike guaifenesin which is an expectorant. Pseudoephedrine is a decongestant and loratadine an antihistamine. Technicians must monitor pseudoephedrine sales due to Combat Methamphetamine Epidemic Act restrictions.
Q72. Answer: A
Explanation: Metronidazole causes a disulfiram-like reaction with alcohol, producing nausea, flushing, and vomiting. Patients must abstain from alcohol during therapy and for 48 hours after completion. Doxycycline, azithromycin, and cephalexin lack this reaction. Technicians should apply auxiliary labels highlighting this contraindication.
Q73. Answer: C
Explanation: Quetiapine is an atypical antipsychotic with serotonin and dopamine receptor antagonism, producing fewer extrapyramidal side effects than typical agents. Haloperidol, chlorpromazine, and fluphenazine are first-generation antipsychotics associated with higher movement disorder risk. Monitoring for metabolic effects like weight gain is required.
Q74. Answer: B
Explanation: Albuterol provides rapid bronchodilation during asthma attacks by activating beta-2 receptors in airway smooth muscle. Salmeterol and formoterol are long-acting agents, and tiotropium is an anticholinergic. Technicians instruct patients on proper inhaler priming and use for effective symptom relief.
Q75. Answer: C
Explanation: Levothyroxine is synthetic T_4 replacing deficient thyroid hormone. Methimazole and propylthiouracil suppress hormone production in hyperthyroidism, while prednisone is unrelated. Patients should take levothyroxine on an empty stomach with water and avoid calcium or iron within four hours to ensure proper absorption.
Q76. Answer: A
Explanation: Fluoxetine, an SSRI, increases serotonin levels and can cause serotonin syndrome if combined with MAOIs or other serotonergic drugs. Bupropion lacks serotonergic activity, while trazodone and mirtazapine act differently. A two-week washout between classes prevents this potentially life-threatening interaction.
Q77. Answer: A
Explanation: Heparin enhances antithrombin's inhibition of clotting factors IIa and Xa, preventing thrombus formation. Warfarin inhibits vitamin K synthesis, while apixaban and dabigatran act directly on clotting enzymes. Heparin requires monitoring of activated partial thromboplastin time (aPTT) for dose adjustment.

Q78. Answer: B
Explanation: Tetracycline binds calcium in dairy products, reducing absorption and effectiveness. Azithromycin, metronidazole, and clindamycin are unaffected. Technicians should counsel patients to avoid milk, крайней antacids, or iron within two hours of tetracycline dosing to preserve therapeutic levels.
Q79. Answer: B
Explanation: Allopurinol inhibits xanthine oxidase, lowering uric acid formation and preventing gout attacks. Colchicine treats acute pain but not prevention, naproxen reduces inflammation, and prednisone manages severe flare-ups. Consistent hydration and dose titration minimize renal stone risk.
Q80. Answer: A
Explanation: Fluticasone nasal spray reduces nasal inflammation and congestion in allergic rhinitis. Loratadine is an oral antihistamine, pseudoephedrine a decongestant, and montelukast a leukotriene blocker. Proper nasal spray technique improves symptom control while minimizing systemic absorption and side effects.
Q81. Answer: B
Explanation: Amoxicillin is a broad-spectrum beta-lactam antibiotic in the penicillin class, inhibiting bacterial cell wall synthesis. Macrolides inhibit protein synthesis, fluoroquinolones disrupt DNA replication, and tetracyclines bind ribosomal subunits. Recognizing antibiotic classes helps technicians prevent therapeutic duplication and identify allergy cross-sensitivity.
Q82. Answer: B
Explanation: Naloxegol is a peripherally acting opioid antagonist that relieves constipation without affecting central analgesia. Docusate and senna are stool softeners and stimulants, while lactulose treats hepatic encephalopathy. Awareness of targeted constipation therapy ensures proper selection in patients on chronic opioid regimens.
Q83. Answer: B
Explanation: Glipizide stimulates pancreatic beta cells to secrete insulin, characteristic of sulfonylureas. Metformin is a biguanide, sitagliptin a DPP-4 inhibitor, and pioglitazone a thiazolidinedione. Monitoring for hypoglycemia is essential, particularly in elderly or renal-impaired patients, to ensure safe glucose control.
Q84. Answer: B
Explanation: Carbidopa/Levodopa combines a dopamine precursor with a decarboxylase inhibitor to enhance CNS dopamine levels. Benztropine is anticholinergic, ropinirole is a dopamine agonist, and selegiline inhibits MAO-B. The combination minimizes peripheral conversion and nausea while optimizing motor control.
Q85. Answer: A
Explanation: Duloxetine, an SNRI, reduces neuropathic pain by enhancing serotonergic and noradrenergic transmission. Lorazepam and clonazepam are benzodiazepines, while paroxetine is an SSRI for depression. Technicians should counsel patients about delayed onset and monitor for blood pressure or mood changes.
Q86. Answer: C
Explanation: Insulin glargine provides steady basal insulin release lasting up to 24 hours, preventing fasting hyperglycemia. Aspart and lispro are rapid-acting, while regular insulin is short-acting. Technicians emphasize consistent timing and avoidance of mixing glargine with other insulin types in the same syringe.
Q87. Answer: A
Explanation: Fibrates such as gemfibrozil activate peroxisome proliferator-activated receptors (PPARs), reducing triglycerides and raising HDL. Statins primarily lower LDL cholesterol, while ACE inhibitors and

ARBs target hypertension. Combining fibrates with statins increases myopathy risk, requiring careful monitoring.

Q88. Answer: B

Explanation: Misoprostol, a prostaglandin analog, protects gastric mucosa and counteracts NSAID-induced ulceration. Sucralfate coats existing ulcers, omeprazole suppresses acid, and ranitidine is an H_2 blocker. Misoprostol is contraindicated in pregnancy due to uterine stimulation, requiring technician verification for female patients.

Q89. Answer: A

Explanation: Trazodone acts as a serotonin receptor antagonist and weak reuptake inhibitor, commonly used for depression and insomnia. Sertraline is an SSRI, venlafaxine an SNRI, and bupropion a dopamine–norepinephrine reuptake inhibitor. Its sedative profile makes it useful for nighttime dosing in depressed patients.

Q90. Answer: B

Explanation: Cephalexin is a first-generation cephalosporin that inhibits bacterial cell wall synthesis. Doxycycline is a tetracycline, levofloxacin a fluoroquinolone, and erythromycin a macrolide. Cephalosporins are effective for skin and soft tissue infections, with minimal cross-allergy risk for most penicillin-allergic patients.

Q91. Answer: A

Explanation: Clonidine reduces sympathetic outflow by stimulating central alpha-2 receptors, lowering blood pressure. Doxazosin blocks peripheral alpha-1 receptors, labetalol adds alpha-blockade, and propranolol is a beta-blocker. Abrupt discontinuation of clonidine can cause rebound hypertension, requiring gradual dose tapering.

Q92. Answer: A

Explanation: Warfarin inhibits vitamin K epoxide reductase, preventing activation of clotting factors II, VII, IX, and X. Heparin enhances antithrombin activity, while apixaban and rivaroxaban directly inhibit Factor Xa. Regular INR monitoring ensures therapeutic effectiveness and safety during warfarin therapy.

Q93. Answer: B

Explanation: Lisinopril inhibits the angiotensin-converting enzyme, decreasing angiotensin II and lowering blood pressure. Losartan blocks angiotensin II receptors, amlodipine blocks calcium channels, and metoprolol blocks beta receptors. ACE inhibitors also reduce proteinuria in diabetic nephropathy, making them first-line for hypertension with kidney involvement.

Q94. Answer: B

Explanation: Buspirone is a non-benzodiazepine anxiolytic that acts on serotonin receptors without sedation or dependency risk. Alprazolam, lorazepam, and diazepam are benzodiazepines with CNS depressant effects. Buspirone requires several weeks for onset, making adherence crucial for therapeutic benefit.

Q95. Answer: B

Explanation: Allopurinol inhibits xanthine oxidase, decreasing uric acid production to prevent gout attacks. Colchicine treats acute flares, naproxen is an NSAID for inflammation, and prednisone is for severe pain management. Consistent hydration and renal dose adjustment are necessary to prevent toxicity.

Q96. Answer: B

Explanation: Montelukast blocks leukotriene receptors, reducing airway inflammation and bronchoconstriction in asthma and allergic rhinitis. Albuterol is a beta-2 agonist, fluticasone a corticosteroid, and tiotropium an anticholinergic. Montelukast is taken daily at night for maintenance, not for acute relief.

Q97. Answer: B

Explanation: Methylphenidate increases dopamine and norepinephrine levels, improving attention and impulse control in ADHD. Atomoxetine is non-stimulant, clonidine is adjunctive, and bupropion is off-label. Technicians should monitor controlled substance regulations and advise early refills due to Schedule II status.

Q98. Answer: B

Explanation: Acetaminophen reduces fever and pain by inhibiting central prostaglandin synthesis without anti-inflammatory effects. Ibuprofen and naproxen are NSAIDs, while tramadol is a weak opioid agonist. Overdose can cause hepatotoxicity, so technicians must warn patients to avoid combining with other acetaminophen-containing products.

Q99. Answer: A

Explanation: Clopidogrel inhibits platelet aggregation by blocking ADP receptors, preventing clot formation after stent placement or stroke. Warfarin and apixaban are anticoagulants affecting clotting factors, while heparin enhances antithrombin. Patients should report bleeding signs and avoid concurrent NSAIDs.

Q100. Answer: B

Explanation: Flumazenil competitively inhibits benzodiazepine binding at GABA receptors, reversing sedation and respiratory depression. Naloxone reverses opioids, atropine treats bradycardia, and acetylcysteine is for acetaminophen toxicity. Flumazenil should be administered cautiously to avoid seizures in long-term benzodiazepine users.

Questions (101-200)

Q101. Which of these antibiotics is used for acne and can cause tooth discoloration?

A. Amoxicillin
B. Doxycycline
C. Azithromycin
D. Cephalexin

Q102. Which of the following medications is used to treat seizures and also for trigeminal neuralgia?

A. Valproic acid
B. Carbamazepine
C. Phenytoin
D. Gabapentin

Q103. Which drug is a long-acting muscarinic antagonist used in COPD maintenance therapy?

A. Ipratropium
B. Tiotropium
C. Albuterol
D. Formoterol

Q104. Which of the following medications is used for insomnia and acts on melatonin receptors?

A. Eszopiclone
B. Zolpidem
C. Ramelteon
D. Trazodone

Q105. Which drug class does hydrochlorothiazide belong to?

A. Loop diuretics
B. Thiazide diuretics
C. Potassium-sparing diuretics
D. Osmotic diuretics

Q106. Which of the following medications is a calcium supplement used in osteoporosis prevention?

A. Alendronate
B. Ergocalciferol
C. Calcitonin
D. Calcium carbonate

Q107. Which medication is an NMDA receptor antagonist used for moderate Alzheimer's disease?

A. Donepezil
B. Memantine
C. Rivastigmine
D. Galantamine

Q108. Which of these medications is used as a topical antifungal for athlete's foot?

A. Clindamycin
B. Nystatin
C. Terbinafine
D. Metronidazole

Q109. Which medication is a benzodiazepine used for short-term anxiety relief?

A. Buspirone
B. Diazepam
C. Escitalopram
D. Sertraline

Q110. Which drug is an SSRI antidepressant also used for obsessive-compulsive disorder (OCD)?

A. Fluoxetine
B. Duloxetine
C. Amitriptyline
D. Bupropion

Q111. Which of these medications is a proton pump inhibitor used for GERD?

A. Famotidine
B. Omeprazole
C. Sucralfate
D. Metoclopramide

Q112. Which anticoagulant is given by subcutaneous injection for DVT prophylaxis?

A. Warfarin
B. Heparin
C. Enoxaparin
D. Dabigatran

Q113. Which medication acts as an antiemetic by blocking dopamine receptors?

A. Ondansetron
B. Metoclopramide
C. Promethazine
D. Diphenhydramine

Q114. Which of these medications is a bisphosphonate for osteoporosis treatment?

A. Raloxifene
B. Alendronate
C. Calcitonin
D. Teriparatide

Q115. Which drug is a selective serotonin reuptake inhibitor (SSRI) with the fewest drug interactions?

A. Paroxetine
B. Fluoxetine
C. Escitalopram
D. Sertraline

Q116. Which drug is used to treat attention deficit hyperactivity disorder (ADHD) as a non-stimulant?

A. Methylphenidate
B. Dextroamphetamine
C. Atomoxetine
D. Lisdexamfetamine

Q117. Which of the following is a serotonin receptor agonist used for acute migraine treatment?

A. Sumatriptan
B. Propranolol
C. Topiramate
D. Ergotamine

Q118. Which medication is a corticosteroid used topically for inflammation?

A. Triamcinolone
B. Hydrocodone
C. Loratadine
D. Clotrimazole

Q119. Which of these medications is an opioid analgesic combined with acetaminophen?

A. Tramadol
B. Hydrocodone/APAP
C. Codeine

D. Morphine

Q120. Which of these medications is an H_2 blocker that decreases stomach acid?

A. Omeprazole

B. Sucralfate

C. Famotidine

D. Misoprostol

Q121. Which of the following medications is a stimulant used for narcolepsy?

A. Zolpidem

B. Modafinil

C. Lorazepam

D. Clonidine

Q122. Which of these medications is an antifungal used to treat oral candidiasis?

A. Fluconazole

B. Nystatin

C. Terbinafine

D. Acyclovir

Q123. Which medication is a beta-blocker also used in migraine prevention?

A. Atenolol

B. Propranolol

C. Metoprolol

D. Bisoprolol

Q124. Which of these medications is a selective estrogen receptor modulator (SERM)?

A. Alendronate

B. Raloxifene

C. Calcitonin

D. Teriparatide

Q125. Which of the following medications is used to treat overactive bladder by antimuscarinic action?

A. Oxybutynin

B. Finasteride

C. Tamsulosin

D. Phenazopyridine

Q126. Which of these medications is used to manage alcohol dependence?

A. Naltrexone

B. Naloxone

C. Methadone

D. Diazepam

Q127. Which of these medications is a corticosteroid used to prevent asthma exacerbations?

A. Prednisone

B. Albuterol

C. Fluticasone

D. Montelukast

Q128. Which antiepileptic medication can cause gum overgrowth?

A. Phenytoin

B. Carbamazepine

C. Valproic acid

D. Levetiracetam

Q129. Which antibiotic is commonly prescribed for urinary tract infections?

A. Amoxicillin
B. Ciprofloxacin
C. Clindamycin
D. Azithromycin

Q130. Which of the following is a monoclonal antibody used for rheumatoid arthritis?
A. Methotrexate
B. Adalimumab
C. Prednisone
D. Leflunomide

Q131. Which antidepressant is also approved for fibromyalgia pain?
A. Fluoxetine
B. Duloxetine
C. Bupropion
D. Paroxetine

Q132. Which of the following drugs is a benzodiazepine used as an anticonvulsant?
A. Diazepam
B. Lorazepam
C. Clonazepam
D. Alprazolam

Q133. Which of these drugs is a loop diuretic used for pulmonary edema?
A. Furosemide
B. Hydrochlorothiazide
C. Spironolactone
D. Torsemide

Q134. Which antipsychotic is least likely to cause extrapyramidal side effects?
A. Haloperidol
B. Risperidone
C. Quetiapine
D. Fluphenazine

Q135. Which of these medications is used to lower LDL cholesterol by inhibiting intestinal absorption?
A. Ezetimibe
B. Atorvastatin
C. Gemfibrozil
D. Niacin

Q136. Which drug is an antiemetic that blocks histamine and dopamine receptors?
A. Promethazine
B. Ondansetron
C. Metoclopramide
D. Diphenhydramine

Q137. Which of these medications is used to prevent seizures in eclampsia?
A. Lorazepam
B. Phenytoin
C. Magnesium sulfate
D. Valproic acid

Q138. Which medication is an antifungal that inhibits ergosterol synthesis?
A. Fluconazole
B. Acyclovir
C. Metronidazole

D. Clindamycin

Q139. Which of these medications is a beta-2 agonist used for acute asthma attacks?

A. Formoterol

B. Salmeterol

C. Albuterol

D. Montelukast

Q140. Which of the following drugs is an opioid analgesic also used for cough suppression?

A. Hydrocodone

B. Morphine

C. Oxycodone

D. Methadone

Q141. Which of the following medications is used for opioid withdrawal symptom relief?

A. Buprenorphine

B. Naloxone

C. Methadone

D. Clonidine

Q142. Which of these medications is an SSRI used for panic disorder?

A. Fluoxetine

B. Amitriptyline

C. Duloxetine

D. Trazodone

Q143. Which medication acts as an antidote for heparin overdose?

A. Protamine sulfate

B. Vitamin K

C. Atropine

D. Flumazenil

Q144. Which of these drugs is an anticonvulsant also used for migraine prevention?

A. Levetiracetam

B. Valproic acid

C. Phenytoin

D. Lamotrigine

Q145. Which of these drugs is an antiarrhythmic that may cause pulmonary toxicity?

A. Amiodarone

B. Digoxin

C. Verapamil

D. Metoprolol

Q146. Which medication is used as an expectorant to relieve chest congestion?

A. Guaifenesin

B. Dextromethorphan

C. Loratadine

D. Pseudoephedrine

Q147. Which medication is a potassium-sparing diuretic and aldosterone antagonist?

A. Hydrochlorothiazide

B. Furosemide

C. Spironolactone

D. Torsemide

Q148. Which of the following drugs is used as an oral antiplatelet agent after myocardial infarction?

A. Warfarin

B. Clopidogrel
C. Apixaban
D. Dabigatran

Q149. Which of the following is an anticholinergic bronchodilator used in COPD?
A. Ipratropium
B. Albuterol
C. Formoterol
D. Salmeterol

Q150. Which of the following antibiotics belongs to the aminoglycoside class?
A. Gentamicin
B. Azithromycin
C. Ceftriaxone
D. Levofloxacin

Q151. Which of these medications is a beta-blocker used for glaucoma?
A. Latanoprost
B. Pilocarpine
C. Brimonidine
D. Timolol

Q152. Which drug is an anticonvulsant that can cause Stevens–Johnson syndrome?
A. Lamotrigine
B. Phenytoin
C. Carbamazepine
D. Valproic acid

Q153. Which medication is a thiazolidinedione used to increase insulin sensitivity?
A. Pioglitazone
B. Glipizide
C. Metformin
D. Sitagliptin

Q154. Which of these medications is an antipsychotic also approved for bipolar depression?
A. Clozapine
B. Risperidone
C. Quetiapine
D. Haloperidol

Q155. Which of the following drugs is used to treat bacterial vaginosis?
A. Fluconazole
B. Metronidazole
C. Miconazole
D. Nystatin

Q156. Which medication is a serotonin-norepinephrine reuptake inhibitor used for depression?
A. Escitalopram
B. Duloxetine
C. Bupropion
D. Trazodone

Q157. Which antipsychotic is associated with the highest risk of metabolic syndrome?
A. Aripiprazole
B. Clozapine
C. Ziprasidone
D. Risperidone

Q158. Which of these drugs is a non-steroidal anti-inflammatory with COX-2 selectivity?
A. Ibuprofen
B. Naproxen
C. Celecoxib
D. Ketorolac
Q159. Which of the following medications is an antitussive that acts on the cough center in the medulla?
A. Guaifenesin
B. Dextromethorphan
C. Loratadine
D. Pseudoephedrine
Q160. Which of these drugs is a carbonic anhydrase inhibitor used for glaucoma?
A. Dorzolamide
B. Latanoprost
C. Timolol
D. Brimonidine
Q161. Which of the following is a topical antibiotic commonly used for skin infections?
A. Mupirocin
B. Clindamycin
C. Ciprofloxacin
D. Metronidazole
Q162. Which medication is an anticoagulant that does not require INR monitoring?
A. Warfarin
B. Apixaban
C. Heparin
D. Enoxaparin
Q163. Which of these medications is a dopamine agonist used in Parkinson's disease?
A. Selegiline
B. Carbidopa/Levodopa
C. Ropinirole
D. Amantadine
Q164. Which drug is an ACE inhibitor commonly prescribed for heart failure?
A. Metoprolol
B. Lisinopril
C. Losartan
D. Amlodipine
Q165. Which of the following medications is a beta-lactam antibiotic with a beta-lactamase inhibitor?
A. Amoxicillin-clavulanate
B. Ceftriaxone
C. Doxycycline
D. Azithromycin
Q166. Which of these medications is an antimalarial that can cause retinal toxicity?
A. Metronidazole
B. Chloroquine
C. Doxycycline
D. Isoniazid
Q167. Which drug is an HMG-CoA reductase inhibitor used to lower cholesterol?
A. Gemfibrozil

B. Atorvastatin
C. Ezetimibe
D. Niacin

Q168. Which antibiotic is known for causing hearing loss and nephrotoxicity?
A. Vancomycin
B. Gentamicin
C. Linezolid
D. Cefepime

Q169. Which of these medications is used for type 2 diabetes and may cause bladder cancer risk with long-term use?
A. Metformin
B. Pioglitazone
C. Glipizide
D. Sitagliptin

Q170. Which of the following is an alpha-blocker used to treat hypertension?
A. Terazosin
B. Amlodipine
C. Lisinopril
D. Furosemide

Q171. Which antiemetic blocks serotonin (5-HT_3) receptors?
A. Promethazine
B. Ondansetron
C. Metoclopramide
D. Diphenhydramine

Q172. Which of these medications is a macrolide antibiotic?
A. Erythromycin
B. Cefdinir
C. Doxycycline
D. Ciprofloxacin

Q173. Which drug is a direct thrombin inhibitor used for stroke prevention in atrial fibrillation?
A. Apixaban
B. Dabigatran
C. Rivaroxaban
D. Warfarin

Q174. Which of the following medications is an inhaled corticosteroid combined with a long-acting beta agonist (LABA)?
A. Advair Diskus®
B. Ventolin®
C. Singulair®
D. Spiriva®

Q175. Which antibiotic is contraindicated in children due to risk of tooth discoloration and bone effects?
A. Azithromycin
B. Doxycycline
C. Amoxicillin
D. Cefdinir

Q176. Which medication is a proton pump inhibitor used for peptic ulcer disease?
A. Pantoprazole

B. Sucralfate
C. Ranitidine
D. Famotidine

Q177. Which of these drugs is a corticosteroid nasal spray used for allergic rhinitis?
A. Fluticasone
B. Loratadine
C. Montelukast
D. Oxymetazoline

Q178. Which of the following antidiabetic drugs can cause lactic acidosis as a rare side effect?
A. Glipizide
B. Metformin
C. Pioglitazone
D. Sitagliptin

Q179. Which of these medications is a leukotriene receptor antagonist used in asthma prevention?
A. Albuterol
B. Montelukast
C. Salmeterol
D. Theophylline

Q180. Which of the following is an H_2 blocker used for GERD?
A. Omeprazole
B. Sucralfate
C. Famotidine
D. Misoprostol

Q181. Which of these medications is a proton pump inhibitor used for ulcer prevention?
A. Famotidine
B. Pantoprazole
C. Sucralfate
D. Ranitidine

Q182. Which of the following medications is a dopamine antagonist used as an antipsychotic?
A. Haloperidol
B. Lorazepam
C. Clonidine
D. Carbamazepine

Q183. Which of these medications is used as an antidote for acetaminophen overdose?
A. Atropine
B. Acetylcysteine
C. Flumazenil
D. Naloxone

Q184. Which drug is an estrogen used for hormone replacement therapy in postmenopausal women?
A. Estradiol
B. Medroxyprogesterone
C. Finasteride
D. Clomiphene

Q185. Which of these medications is a biguanide antidiabetic agent?
A. Pioglitazone
B. Glipizide
C. Metformin
D. Sitagliptin

Q186. Which of the following antibiotics is associated with tendon rupture risk?
A. Ciprofloxacin
B. Amoxicillin
C. Doxycycline
D. Azithromycin
Q187. Which of these medications is an opioid antagonist used for opioid overdose?
A. Methadone
B. Naloxone
C. Buprenorphine
D. Clonidine
Q188. Which of the following drugs is used for thyroid hormone replacement therapy?
A. Methimazole
B. Levothyroxine
C. Propylthiouracil
D. Liothyronine
Q189. Which of these medications is an ACE inhibitor combined with a thiazide diuretic?
A. Lisinopril/HCTZ
B. Losartan/HCTZ
C. Amlodipine/Benazepril
D. Valsartan/HCTZ
Q190. Which drug is a non-opioid analgesic that acts centrally and peripherally?
A. Ibuprofen
B. Naproxen
C. Acetaminophen
D. Aspirin
Q191. Which of these medications is a beta-blocker with intrinsic sympathomimetic activity?
A. Pindolol
B. Metoprolol
C. Atenolol
D. Propranolol
Q192. Which of the following medications is an anticholinergic used for motion sickness?
A. Diphenhydramine
B. Meclizine
C. Scopolamine
D. Promethazine
Q193. Which of these antibiotics is used to treat MRSA infections?
A. Amoxicillin
B. Vancomycin
C. Ceftriaxone
D. Azithromycin
Q194. Which of these drugs is an antihypertensive that can cause a persistent dry cough?
A. Lisinopril
B. Losartan
C. Amlodipine
D. Metoprolol
Q195. Which drug is an SSRI antidepressant also approved for premature ejaculation?
A. Paroxetine
B. Fluoxetine

C. Sertraline
D. Citalopram
Q196. Which of these medications is a leukotriene receptor antagonist?
A. Montelukast
B. Albuterol
C. Fluticasone
D. Tiotropium
Q197. Which of these medications is a stool softener used to prevent constipation?
A. Senna
B. Polyethylene glycol
C. Docusate sodium
D. Bisacodyl
Q198. Which medication is an alpha-1 blocker used for benign prostatic hyperplasia (BPH)?
A. Finasteride
B. Tamsulosin
C. Dutasteride
D. Oxybutynin
Q199. Which of these medications is a vitamin K antagonist used for anticoagulation?
A. Heparin
B. Warfarin
C. Apixaban
D. Dabigatran
Q200. Which of the following medications is an opioid used to manage chronic pain?
A. Tramadol
B. Morphine
C. Ibuprofen
D. Acetaminophen

Answer key and Explanation (101-200)

Q101. Answer: B

Explanation: Doxycycline, a tetracycline antibiotic, binds calcium in teeth and bones, leading to discoloration in children or long-term use. Amoxicillin, azithromycin, and cephalexin lack this side effect. Technicians must caution patients to avoid dairy and take with water to improve absorption and minimize esophageal irritation.

Q102. Answer: B

Explanation: Carbamazepine stabilizes neuronal membranes by inhibiting sodium channels, effectively treating seizures and trigeminal neuralgia pain. Valproic acid treats generalized seizures, phenytoin prevents tonic–clonic episodes, and gabapentin alleviates neuropathy. Regular CBC monitoring is necessary due to carbamazepine's hematologic side effect risk.

Q103. Answer: B

Explanation: Tiotropium provides 24-hour bronchodilation by blocking muscarinic receptors in airway smooth muscle. Ipratropium is shorter-acting, albuterol is a beta-2 agonist for acute relief, and formoterol is a long-acting beta agonist. Proper inhaler use ensures optimal lung deposition and symptom control.

Q104. Answer: C

Explanation: Ramelteon selectively activates melatonin receptors MT_1 and MT_2 to regulate circadian rhythm without dependency risk. Eszopiclone and zolpidem act on GABA receptors, while trazodone is an antidepressant with sedative effects. Ramelteon is not controlled, making it safer for chronic use.

Q105. Answer: B

Explanation: Hydrochlorothiazide increases sodium and water excretion in the distal convoluted tubule, lowering blood pressure. Loop diuretics act in the loop of Henle, potassium-sparing agents conserve potassium, and osmotic diuretics alter osmolarity. Monitoring electrolytes prevents hypokalemia and dehydration during therapy.

Q106. Answer: D

Explanation: Calcium carbonate provides elemental calcium essential for bone formation and maintenance. Alendronate is a bisphosphonate, ergocalciferol is vitamin D_2, and calcitonin regulates calcium metabolism. Calcium supplements are best taken with meals to enhance absorption and minimize gastrointestinal side effects.

Q107. Answer: B

Explanation: Memantine blocks NMDA receptors to reduce excitotoxicity and slow cognitive decline in Alzheimer's disease. Donepezil, rivastigmine, and galantamine inhibit acetylcholinesterase to enhance cholinergic transmission. Combining memantine with donepezil provides synergistic effects in advanced disease stages.

Q108. Answer: C

Explanation: Terbinafine inhibits squalene epoxidase, disrupting fungal cell membranes, and is effective for tinea infections like athlete's foot. Nystatin treats Candida, clindamycin targets bacteria, and metronidazole is for anaerobes. Advise patients to continue therapy for full duration to prevent recurrence.

Q109. Answer: B

Explanation: Diazepam enhances GABA neurotransmission, producing rapid anxiolytic and muscle relaxant effects. Buspirone is non-sedating but slower-acting, while escitalopram and sertraline are antidepressants. Benzodiazepines are controlled substances requiring strict refill monitoring and caution for dependence with prolonged use.

Q110. Answer: A

Explanation: Fluoxetine increases serotonin in synapses and effectively treats depression, anxiety, and OCD. Duloxetine is an SNRI for pain and depression, amitriptyline is a TCA, and bupropion lacks serotonergic activity. Technicians should caution about delayed onset and risk of serotonin syndrome with concurrent serotonergic drugs.

Q111. Answer: B

Explanation: Omeprazole inhibits gastric H^+/K^+-ATPase, providing long-term acid suppression in GERD. Famotidine blocks H_2 receptors, sucralfate coats ulcers, and metoclopramide enhances gastric motility. PPIs should be taken 30–60 minutes before meals for maximum efficacy and to prevent rebound acid hypersecretion.

Q112. Answer: C

Explanation: Enoxaparin, a low-molecular-weight heparin, is injected subcutaneously to prevent deep vein thrombosis. Warfarin is oral, heparin is IV or subcutaneous but less specific, and dabigatran is oral. Proper injection technique and avoidance of rubbing the site minimize bruising.

Q113. Answer: B

Explanation: Metoclopramide blocks dopamine receptors in the chemoreceptor trigger zone, reducing nausea and enhancing gastric motility. Ondansetron blocks serotonin, promethazine blocks histamine, and diphenhydramine is mainly sedative. Long-term use can cause extrapyramidal symptoms, requiring technician awareness of duration limits.

Q114. Answer: B

Explanation: Alendronate inhibits osteoclast-mediated bone resorption, strengthening bones and reducing fracture risk. Raloxifene is a SERM, calcitonin regulates calcium, and teriparatide stimulates bone formation. Patients should take alendronate with water and remain upright for 30 minutes to prevent esophageal irritation.

Q115. Answer: C

Explanation: Escitalopram has minimal CYP450 interactions, making it safer for polypharmacy patients. Paroxetine and fluoxetine inhibit multiple hepatic enzymes, increasing drug interaction risk, while sertraline has intermediate potential. Escitalopram's favorable safety profile makes it a preferred SSRI for first-line depression treatment.

Q116. Answer: C

Explanation: Atomoxetine inhibits norepinephrine reuptake, improving focus without stimulant properties. Methylphenidate, dextroamphetamine, and lisdexamfetamine are controlled stimulants. Atomoxetine requires weeks for effect and can cause liver injury or mood changes, so technicians must emphasize adherence and monitoring.

Q117. Answer: A

Explanation: Sumatriptan activates $5\text{-HT}_1B/_1D$ receptors, causing cranial vasoconstriction and relieving migraine pain. Propranolol prevents migraines, topiramate is a prophylactic anticonvulsant, and ergotamine has similar but less selective action. Patients must avoid repeated dosing within 24 hours to prevent vasospasm.

Q118. Answer: A

Explanation: Triamcinolone reduces local inflammation by suppressing immune responses in skin disorders. Hydrocodone is an opioid, loratadine an antihistamine, and clotrimazole an antifungal. Technicians should advise applying a thin layer to affected areas and avoiding occlusive dressings unless directed.

Q119. Answer: B

Explanation: Hydrocodone/APAP combines an opioid with acetaminophen for synergistic pain relief. Tramadol is a weak opioid agonist, codeine is milder, and morphine is stronger and used alone. Patients must avoid additional acetaminophen products to prevent hepatotoxicity and monitor for drowsiness.

Q120. Answer: C

Explanation: Famotidine competitively inhibits histamine H_2 receptors on gastric parietal cells, reducing acid production. Omeprazole is a PPI, sucralfate forms a protective barrier, and misoprostol is a prostaglandin analog. Famotidine is effective for short-term heartburn and ulcer therapy with minimal side effects.

Q121. Answer: B

Explanation: Modafinil promotes wakefulness by influencing dopamine and orexin pathways, treating narcolepsy and shift work sleep disorder. Zolpidem induces sleep, lorazepam is an anxiolytic, and clonidine lowers blood pressure. Modafinil has lower abuse potential than amphetamines but requires prescription monitoring.

Q122. Answer: B

Explanation: Nystatin binds fungal cell membrane ergosterol, causing leakage and death, ideal for oral candidiasis. Fluconazole treats systemic fungal infections, terbinafine targets dermatophytes, and acyclovir is antiviral. Patients should swish and retain nystatin suspension before swallowing for maximum local effect.

Q123. Answer: B

Explanation: Propranolol, a nonselective beta-blocker, is effective for migraine prophylaxis due to its vasodilatory stabilization. Atenolol, metoprolol, and bisoprolol are cardioselective and mainly antihypertensives. Technicians should verify proper indication and monitor for fatigue, dizziness, and bradycardia in long-term users.

Q124. Answer: B

Explanation: Raloxifene acts as an estrogen agonist in bone and antagonist in breast tissue, reducing osteoporosis risk and breast cancer incidence. Alendronate is a bisphosphonate, calcitonin regulates calcium, and teriparatide stimulates bone formation. It may increase venous thromboembolism risk, warranting caution.

Q125. Answer: A

Explanation: Oxybutynin blocks muscarinic receptors in bladder smooth muscle, reducing urge incontinence. Finasteride and tamsulosin treat BPH via hormonal and alpha-adrenergic pathways, while phenazopyridine relieves urinary discomfort. Dry mouth and constipation are common side effects needing patient counseling.

Q126. Answer: A

Explanation: Naltrexone blocks opioid receptors, reducing the rewarding effects of alcohol consumption. Naloxone reverses opioid overdose, methadone treats opioid dependence, and diazepam manages acute withdrawal anxiety. Oral or injectable naltrexone requires liver function monitoring due to potential hepatotoxicity.

Q127. Answer: C

Explanation: Fluticasone is an inhaled corticosteroid reducing airway inflammation for asthma maintenance. Prednisone is systemic for acute flare-ups, albuterol is a rescue bronchodilator, and montelukast blocks leukotrienes. Rinsing mouth post-inhalation prevents oral thrush, an important technician counseling point.

Q128. Answer: A

Explanation: Phenytoin causes gingival hyperplasia due to altered collagen metabolism. Carbamazepine may cause blood dyscrasias, valproic acid hepatotoxicity, and levetiracetam behavioral changes. Dental hygiene reinforcement is essential to minimize this adverse effect during long-term therapy.

Q129. Answer: B

Explanation: Ciprofloxacin, a fluoroquinolone, effectively treats UTIs by inhibiting bacterial DNA gyrase. Amoxicillin is often ineffective due to resistance, clindamycin targets anaerobes, and azithromycin treats respiratory infections. Technicians should caution about tendon injury risk and hydration during treatment.

Q130. Answer: B
Explanation: Adalimumab targets TNF-α, reducing inflammation in rheumatoid arthritis and Crohn's disease. Methotrexate and leflunomide are DMARDs, while prednisone is corticosteroid adjunct therapy. Adalimumab is injected subcutaneously, requiring refrigeration and infection risk counseling for patients.
Q131. Answer: B
Explanation: Duloxetine, an SNRI, enhances serotonin and norepinephrine transmission, effectively treating both depression and fibromyalgia-related pain. Fluoxetine and paroxetine are SSRIs without pain-relief properties, and bupropion lacks serotonergic activity. Duloxetine's dual mechanism offers antidepressant and analgesic benefits, making it ideal for chronic pain management.
Q132. Answer: C
Explanation: Clonazepam increases GABA activity, preventing seizure propagation and treating panic disorder. Diazepam and lorazepam are used acutely, while alprazolam focuses on anxiety. Clonazepam's long half-life aids maintenance therapy but requires caution for dependence and drowsiness.
Q133. Answer: A
Explanation: Furosemide acts on the loop of Henle, causing potent sodium and water excretion, ideal for rapid edema relief. Hydrochlorothiazide is weaker, spironolactone is potassium-sparing, and torsemide is similar but longer-acting. Electrolyte monitoring prevents hypokalemia and dehydration.
Q134. Answer: C
Explanation: Quetiapine's low dopamine receptor affinity reduces extrapyramidal symptoms while effectively treating schizophrenia and bipolar disorder. Haloperidol and fluphenazine are high-risk typical agents, and risperidone carries intermediate risk. Quetiapine's metabolic side effects require monitoring of weight and glucose levels.
Q135. Answer: A
Explanation: Ezetimibe blocks cholesterol absorption in the small intestine, reducing LDL levels. Atorvastatin inhibits cholesterol synthesis, gemfibrozil lowers triglycerides, and niacin raises HDL. Ezetimibe is often combined with statins for additional LDL reduction without increasing muscle toxicity risk.
Q136. Answer: A
Explanation: Promethazine prevents nausea by antagonizing histamine and dopamine receptors in the vomiting center. Ondansetron acts on serotonin receptors, metoclopramide on dopamine, and diphenhydramine mainly causes sedation. Promethazine also treats motion sickness but can cause significant drowsiness.
Q137. Answer: C
Explanation: Magnesium sulfate depresses neuromuscular transmission, preventing seizures in preeclampsia and eclampsia. Lorazepam and phenytoin are ineffective for this indication, and valproic acid is teratogenic. Technicians must ensure correct IV dosing and monitor for respiratory depression.
Q138. Answer: A
Explanation: Fluconazole blocks fungal cytochrome P450 enzymes needed for ergosterol synthesis, disrupting cell membranes. Acyclovir treats viral infections, metronidazole targets anaerobes, and clindamycin covers Gram-positive bacteria. Fluconazole is first-line for systemic and mucocutaneous fungal infections.
Q139. Answer: C
Explanation: Albuterol provides rapid bronchodilation by stimulating beta-2 receptors, relieving wheezing within minutes. Formoterol and salmeterol are long-acting, while montelukast is preventive. Patients should be counseled on proper inhaler technique and overuse risks causing paradoxical bronchospasm.
Q140. Answer: A

Explanation: Hydrocodone acts on mu-opioid receptors, relieving pain and suppressing cough reflexes. Morphine and oxycodone are stronger analgesics, while methadone is used for opioid maintenance. Technicians should monitor acetaminophen content in combination formulations to prevent liver toxicity.

Q141. Answer: D

Explanation: Clonidine, an alpha-2 agonist, reduces autonomic withdrawal symptoms such as sweating and agitation by lowering sympathetic tone. Buprenorphine and methadone treat dependence directly, while naloxone reverses overdose. Clonidine assists during detoxification but requires monitoring for hypotension and drowsiness.

Q142. Answer: A

Explanation: Fluoxetine increases serotonin levels and treats depression, panic disorder, and OCD. Amitriptyline is a TCA, duloxetine is an SNRI, and trazodone primarily induces sleep. Consistent dosing and gradual tapering prevent withdrawal or serotonin imbalance symptoms in long-term use.

Q143. Answer: A

Explanation: Protamine sulfate neutralizes heparin by binding its acidic groups, reversing anticoagulation. Vitamin K reverses warfarin, atropine treats bradycardia, and flumazenil reverses benzodiazepines. Protamine must be administered slowly to prevent hypotension and allergic reactions, especially in fish-allergic patients.

Q144. Answer: B

Explanation: Valproic acid prevents seizures and migraines by increasing GABA levels. Levetiracetam treats seizures but not migraines, phenytoin is limited to seizure control, and lamotrigine prevents bipolar episodes. Monitoring liver enzymes and platelets ensures early detection of potential hepatotoxicity.

Q145. Answer: A

Explanation: Amiodarone, a class III antiarrhythmic, prolongs repolarization and may cause pulmonary fibrosis with chronic use. Digoxin increases contractility, verapamil is a calcium blocker, and metoprolol is a beta-blocker. Baseline chest X-rays and thyroid monitoring are required for patients on amiodarone.

Q146. Answer: A

Explanation: Guaifenesin thins bronchial secretions, facilitating productive coughs and mucus clearance. Dextromethorphan suppresses cough reflex, loratadine is an antihistamine, and pseudoephedrine is a decongestant. Technicians should encourage hydration for maximum expectorant effectiveness.

Q147. Answer: C

Explanation: Spironolactone inhibits aldosterone in the distal nephron, retaining potassium while excreting sodium and water. Hydrochlorothiazide and furosemide increase potassium loss, while torsemide is a loop diuretic. Monitoring serum potassium is essential to prevent hyperkalemia, especially with ACE inhibitors.

Q148. Answer: B

Explanation: Clopidogrel blocks ADP receptors on platelets, reducing aggregation and clot formation. Warfarin, apixaban, and dabigatran act on clotting factors, not platelets. Clopidogrel prevents re-thrombosis post-stent placement and must be taken consistently to maintain protection.

Q149. Answer: A

Explanation: Ipratropium blocks muscarinic receptors in bronchial smooth muscle, reducing constriction and mucus production. Albuterol is a beta-2 agonist, formoterol and salmeterol are long-acting beta agonists. Ipratropium is often combined with albuterol for dual bronchodilation in COPD therapy.

Q150. Answer: A

Explanation: Gentamicin inhibits bacterial protein synthesis by bindingчок the 30S ribosomal subunit, effective for severe Gram-negative infections. Azithromycin is a macrolide, ceftriaxone a cephalosporin, and levofloxacin a fluoroquinolone. Monitoring renal function and peak/trough levels prevents nephrotoxicity.

Q151. Answer: D
Explanation: Timolol decreases aqueous humor production, reducing intraocular pressure in glaucoma. Pilocarpine increases drainage, brimonidine is an alpha agonist, and latanoprost enhances uveoscleral outflow. Proper drop administration technique avoids systemic beta-blockade side effects such as bradycardia.
Q152. Answer: A
Explanation: Lamotrigine blocks sodium channels and stabilizes mood but carries a black box warning for Stevens–Johnson syndrome, especially during rapid titration. Phenytoin and carbamazepine share this risk, but less commonly. Patients should report rash immediately to prevent severe progression.
Q153. Answer: A
Explanation: Pioglitazone enhances insulin sensitivity via PPAR-γ activation, improving glucose uptake in type 2 diabetes. Glipizide stimulates insulin release, metformin decreases hepatic glucose output, and sitagliptin increases incretin levels. Weight gain and edema are notable adverse effects requiring counseling.
Q154. Answer: C
Explanation: Quetiapine treats schizophrenia, bipolar disorder, and adjunctive depression by modulating serotonin and dopamine receptors. Clozapine is reserved for resistant schizophrenia, risperidone for psychosis, and haloperidol is typical with higher EPS risk. Monitor for metabolic effects such as weight gain.
Q155. Answer: B
Explanation: Metronidazole treats bacterial vaginosis by disrupting bacterial DNA synthesis in anaerobes. Fluconazole and miconazole target fungal infections, while nystatin treats Candida. Patients should avoid alcohol during and 48 hours after therapy to prevent disulfiram-like reactions.
Q156. Answer: B
Explanation: Duloxetine blocks serotonin and norepinephrine reuptake, enhancing mood and relieving neuropathic pain. Escitalopram is an SSRI, bupropion affects dopamine/norepinephrine, and trazodone is mainly sedative. Duloxetine should be tapered to avoid withdrawal and monitored for liver toxicity.
Q157. Answer: B
Explanation: Clozapine significantly increases risk of weight gain, hyperglycemia, and dyslipidemia. Aripiprazole and ziprasidone have lower metabolic risks, while risperidone is intermediate. Technicians should ensure routine metabolic monitoring and reinforce adherence to avoid psychotic relapse.
Q158. Answer: C
Explanation: Celecoxib selectively inhibits COX-2, reducing inflammation while minimizing gastric irritation seen with nonselective NSAIDs. Ibuprofen and naproxen inhibit both COX-1 and COX-2, and ketorolac is for short-term use only. Patients with sulfa allergy should avoid celecoxib.
Q159. Answer: B
Explanation: Dextromethorphan suppresses the cough reflex centrally without opioid effects at normal doses. Guaifenesin loosens mucus, loratadine treats allergies, and pseudoephedrine decongests nasal passages. High doses can cause euphoria and are monitored due to abuse potential.
Q160. Answer: A
Explanation: Dorzolamide decreases aqueous humor production by inhibiting carbonic anhydrase in the ciliary body, lowering intraocular pressure. Latanoprost increases outflow, timolol reduces secretion via beta-blockade, and brimonidine is an alpha agonist. Dorzolamide can cause a bitter taste or eye irritation.
Q161. Answer: A
Explanation: Mupirocin inhibits bacterial protein synthesis and is applied topically for impetigo and other skin infections caused by *Staphylococcus aureus*. Clindamycin can also be topical but is mainly systemic, while ciprofloxacin and metronidazole are oral or IV antibiotics.

Q162. Answer: B
Explanation: Apixaban directly inhibits Factor Xa, providing consistent anticoagulation without INR monitoring. Warfarin requires INR checks due to dietary and drug interactions, while heparin and enoxaparin are injectable. Apixaban's predictable pharmacokinetics simplify outpatient anticoagulant therapy.
Q163. Answer: C
Explanation: Ropinirole stimulates dopamine receptors, alleviating motor symptoms in Parkinson's disease. Carbidopa/Levodopa increases dopamine synthesis, selegiline inhibits its breakdown, and amantadine promotes release. Ropinirole can cause dizziness and sleep attacks, requiring caution in activities like driving.
Q164. Answer: B
Explanation: Lisinopril reduces angiotensin II formation, decreasing vascular resistance and cardiac workload in heart failure. Metoprolol is a beta-blocker, losartan an ARB, and amlodipine a calcium-channel blocker. ACE inhibitors improve survival in systolic dysfunction but may cause cough or hyperkalemia.
Q165. Answer: A
Explanation: Amoxicillin-clavulanate combines a penicillin antibiotic with a beta-lactamase inhibitor to overcome bacterial resistance. Ceftriaxone is a cephalosporin, doxycycline a tetracycline, and azithromycin a macrolide. Technicians should advise taking with food to reduce gastrointestinal upset.
Q166. Answer: B
Explanation: Chloroquine accumulates in retinal tissue, potentially causing irreversible damage with prolonged use. Metronidazole treats anaerobic infections, doxycycline prevents malaria, and isoniazid targets tuberculosis. Regular eye examinations are recommended during long-term chloroquine therapy.
Q167. Answer: B
Explanation: Atorvastatin inhibits HMG-CoA reductase, reducing LDL cholesterol production in the liver. Gemfibrozil lowers triglycerides, ezetimibe blocks absorption, and niacin reduces VLDL secretion. Statins require liver function monitoring and patient education on reporting muscle pain or weakness.
Q168. Answer: B
Explanation: Gentamicin, an aminoglycoside, can cause ototoxicity and nephrotoxicity due to accumulation in renal and auditory cells. Vancomycin shares nephrotoxic potential but not ototoxicity as often. Serum level monitoring is essential to prevent irreversible damage from high trough concentrations.
Q169. Answer: B
Explanation: Pioglitazone, a thiazolidinedione, increases insulin sensitivity but is linked to fluid retention and possible bladder cancer risk. Metformin reduces hepatic glucose production, glipizide stimulates insulin secretion, and sitagliptin enhances incretin activity. Technicians must flag contraindications for heart failure.
Q170. Answer: A
Explanation: Terazosin blocks peripheral alpha-1 receptors, relaxing vascular smooth muscle and reducing blood pressure. Amlodipine is a calcium-channel blocker, lisinopril an ACE inhibitor, and furosemide a diuretic. Terazosin may cause orthostatic hypotension, so patients should rise slowly from sitting positions.
Q171. Answer: B
Explanation: Ondansetron prevents nausea by blocking serotonin receptors in the brain and GI tract. Promethazine and diphenhydramine block histamine, while metoclopramide blocks dopamine. Ondansetron is first-line for chemotherapy- or postoperative-induced nausea and is generally well tolerated.
Q172. Answer: A

Explanation: Erythromycin, a macrolide, inhibits bacterial protein synthesis via the 50S ribosomal subunit. Cefdinir is a cephalosporin, doxycycline a tetracycline, and ciprofloxacin a fluoroquinolone. Macrolides may prolong QT interval, requiring caution in cardiac patients.

Q173. Answer: B

Explanation: Dabigatran directly inhibits thrombin, preventing clot formation in atrial fibrillation. Apixaban and rivaroxaban inhibit Factor Xa, and warfarin blocks vitamin K–dependent clotting factors. Dabigatran capsules must remain in original containers to protect from moisture degradation.

Q174. Answer: A

Explanation: Advair Diskus® combines fluticasone (ICS) and salmeterol (LABA) for asthma and COPD maintenance. Ventolin® contains albuterol for rescue use, Singulair® is montelukast, and Spiriva® is tiotropium. Rinse mouth post-inhalation to prevent oral thrush from steroid residue.

Q175. Answer: B

Explanation: Doxycycline binds calcium, causing permanent tooth discoloration and bone growth inhibition in children under 8 years. Azithromycin, amoxicillin, and cefdinir are safer pediatric options. Technicians should verify patient age before dispensing tetracyclines.

Q176. Answer: A

Explanation: Pantoprazole blocks gastric acid secretion by inhibiting the proton pump, allowing ulcers to heal. Sucralfate coats ulcers, while ranitidine and famotidine are H_2 blockers. Long-term use may lead to vitamin B_{12} deficiency and should be periodically reviewed.

Q177. Answer: A

Explanation: Fluticasone reduces nasal inflammation and allergic symptoms by inhibiting local cytokine release. Loratadine is an antihistamine, montelukast is oral, and oxymetazoline is a short-term decongestant. Regular use provides best results, but overuse may cause nasal dryness.

Q178. Answer: B

Explanation: Metformin reduces hepatic glucose production but can cause lactic acidosis in patients with renal impairment or hypoxia. Glipizide stimulates insulin release, pioglitazone increases sensitivity, and sitagliptin affects incretin levels. Technicians should confirm renal function before dispensing.

Q179. Answer: B

Explanation: Montelukast prevents airway inflammation and bronchoconstriction by blocking leukotriene receptors. Albuterol and salmeterol are bronchodilators, while theophylline relaxes smooth muscle but has narrow safety margins. Montelukast is taken nightly for long-term control, not acute attacks.

Q180. Answer: C

Explanation: Famotidine competitively blocks H_2 receptors in gastric parietal cells, reducing acid secretion and promoting ulcer healing. Omeprazole is a PPI, sucralfate protects ulcers, and misoprostol prevents NSAID-induced gastric injury. Famotidine provides quick relief for mild heartburn symptoms.

Q181. Answer: B

Explanation: Pantoprazole irreversibly inhibits gastric H^+/K^+-ATPase, decreasing acid production and allowing ulcers to heal. Famotidine and ranitidine are H_2 blockers, while sucralfate protects ulcer sites. PPIs should be taken before meals and not used long-term without physician supervision due to rebound acid secretion risk.

Q182. Answer: A

Explanation: Haloperidol blocks dopamine D_2 receptors, managing psychotic symptoms such as hallucinations and agitation. Lorazepam is a benzodiazepine, clonidine lowers blood pressure, and carbamazepine is an anticonvulsant. Haloperidol has a high risk of extrapyramidal symptoms, requiring technician monitoring for side effects.

Q183. Answer: B

Explanation: Acetylcysteine replenishes glutathione stores, neutralizing acetaminophen's toxic metabolite in the liver. Atropine reverses bradycardia, flumazenil reverses benzodiazepines, and naloxone reverses opioids. Prompt administration within 8–10 hours is critical for effectiveness.

Q184. Answer: A

Explanation: Estradiol replaces declining estrogen levels to relieve menopausal symptoms and prevent osteoporosis. Medroxyprogesterone is a progestin, finasteride treats BPH, and clomiphene induces ovulation. Technician counseling should include discussion of thromboembolic risks and proper patch or tablet application.

Q185. Answer: C

Explanation: Metformin decreases hepatic glucose production and increases insulin sensitivity, making it first-line therapy for type 2 diabetes. Pioglitazone enhances insulin sensitivity, glipizide stimulates insulin secretion, and sitagliptin acts on incretin hormones. Gastrointestinal upset and lactic acidosis are rare but serious side effects.

Q186. Answer: A

Explanation: Ciprofloxacin, a fluoroquinolone, can cause tendonitis or tendon rupture, especially in elderly or corticosteroid users. Amoxicillin and azithromycin lack this risk, and doxycycline primarily affects calcium metabolism. Technicians should advise patients to stop use if tendon pain occurs.

Q187. Answer: B

Explanation: Naloxone rapidly displaces opioids from receptors, reversing respiratory depression and sedation. Methadone and buprenorphine are opioid agonists/partial agonists, and clonidine alleviates withdrawal symptoms. Intranasal formulations make naloxone accessible for emergency public use.

Q188. Answer: B

Explanation: Levothyroxine (T_4) replaces deficient thyroid hormone in hypothyroidism. Methimazole and propylthiouracil inhibit thyroid hormone synthesis, while liothyronine is synthetic T_3 used occasionally. Consistent dosing timing and brand selection are crucial to maintain stable thyroid levels.

Q189. Answer: A

Explanation: Lisinopril/HCTZ combines an ACE inhibitor and diuretic for synergistic blood pressure control. Losartan/HCTZ and Valsartan/HCTZ combine ARBs with diuretics, while Amlodipine/Benazepril mixes calcium and ACE blockade. Monitoring electrolytes prevents dehydration or imbalances during therapy.

Q190. Answer: C

Explanation: Acetaminophen reduces pain and fever through central COX inhibition without significant anti-inflammatory effect. Ibuprofen, naproxen, and aspirin inhibit COX peripherally as NSAIDs. Technicians should warn about hepatotoxicity risk with excessive acetaminophen intake from combination products.

Q191. Answer: A

Explanation: Pindolol provides mild beta stimulation while blocking excessive sympathetic activity, useful for patients with bradycardia risk. Metoprolol, atenolol, and propranolol lack this feature. Its unique action minimizes severe heart rate drops while maintaining antihypertensive efficacy.

Q192. Answer: C

Explanation: Scopolamine blocks acetylcholine in the vestibular system, preventing nausea and dizziness from motion sickness. Meclizine and promethazine are antihistamines, while diphenhydramine primarily aids sleep and allergy. Transdermal scopolamine patches are applied behind the ear every three days.

Q193. Answer: B

Explanation: Vancomycin inhibits bacterial cell wall synthesis and is reserved for MRSA and severe Gram-positive infections. Amoxicillin and ceftriaxone are ineffective against MRSA, while azithromycin targets atypical pathogens. Serum level monitoring ensures therapeutic efficacy and minimizes nephrotoxicity.

Q194. Answer: A

Explanation: Lisinopril's inhibition of ACE increases bradykinin levels, causing cough in some patients. Losartan, an ARB, avoids this issue; amlodipine and metoprolol have unrelated mechanisms. Technicians should recommend consulting prescribers about switching to ARBs if cough becomes intolerable.

Q195. Answer: A

Explanation: Paroxetine delays ejaculation by enhancing serotonergic tone while treating depression and anxiety. Fluoxetine, sertraline, and citalopram are also SSRIs but not specifically indicated for this use. Dose adjustments may be needed to minimize sexual side effects in other contexts.

Q196. Answer: A

Explanation: Montelukast blocks leukotriene-mediated inflammation, preventing asthma and allergic rhinitis symptoms. Albuterol is a bronchodilator, fluticasone a corticosteroid, and tiotropium an anticholinergic. Taken nightly, montelukast reduces inflammation and improves long-term respiratory control.

Q197. Answer: C

Explanation: Docusate sodium increases stool moisture, easing passage without stimulating bowel contractions. Senna and bisacodyl are stimulant laxatives, while polyethylene glycol is osmotic. Docusate is ideal for post-surgical or opioid-induced constipation prevention with minimal discomfort.

Q198. Answer: B

Explanation: Tamsulosin relaxes prostate and bladder neck muscles to improve urinary flow in BPH. Finasteride and dutasteride reduce prostate size hormonally, while oxybutynin targets bladder spasms. Orthostatic hypotension and dizziness are common side effects warranting caution during movement.

Q199. Answer: B

Explanation: Warfarin inhibits vitamin K epoxide reductase, preventing activation of clotting factors II, VII, IX, and X. Heparin and newer anticoagulants act directly on thrombin or Factor Xa. Consistent dietary vitamin K intake and INR monitoring are critical for safety.

Q200. Answer: B

Explanation: Morphine binds mu-opioid receptors, providing potent analgesia for chronic or severe pain. Tramadol is weaker and partly serotonergic, while ibuprofen and acetaminophen are non-opioids. Patients must be counseled on constipation prevention, tolerance, and safe storage.

Questions (201-300)

Q201. Which of the following medications is an antihistamine used for allergic rhinitis?

A. Loratadine
B. Dextromethorphan
C. Guaifenesin
D. Montelukast

Q202. Which antibiotic class includes drugs like azithromycin and clarithromycin?

A. Cephalosporins
B. Macrolides
C. Aminoglycosides
D. Tetracyclines

Q203. Which of these medications is a vasodilator used for angina relief?

A. Nitroglycerin
B. Furosemide
C. Metoprolol
D. Verapamil

Q204. Which antiepileptic medication is known for causing gingival hyperplasia?

A. Valproic acid
B. Phenytoin
C. Levetiracetam
D. Topiramate

Q205. Which of the following medications is used to treat generalized anxiety disorder (GAD)?

A. Alprazolam
B. Buspirone
C. Zolpidem
D. Hydroxyzine

Q206. Which of these medications is a bronchodilator used for asthma exacerbations?

A. Albuterol
B. Fluticasone
C. Montelukast
D. Salmeterol

Q207. Which antidepressant also assists in smoking cessation therapy?

A. Paroxetine
B. Bupropion
C. Fluoxetine
D. Sertraline

Q208. Which of the following drugs is used as a mood stabilizer and requires serum monitoring?

A. Risperidone
B. Lithium
C. Haloperidol
D. Quetiapine

Q209. Which medication is an antiarrhythmic that blocks sodium channels?

A. Amiodarone
B. Lidocaine
C. Digoxin
D. Verapamil

Q210. Which of these drugs is an H_2 receptor antagonist used for GERD?

A. Omeprazole
B. Sucralfate
C. Famotidine
D. Misoprostol

Q211. Which of these medications is an antifungal used to treat vaginal candidiasis?
A. Fluconazole
B. Mupirocin
C. Metronidazole
D. Nystatin

Q212. Which antipsychotic is associated with agranulocytosis risk?
A. Risperidone
B. Clozapine
C. Haloperidol
D. Olanzapine

Q213. Which of these medications is used for partial-onset seizures and neuropathic pain?
A. Phenytoin
B. Gabapentin
C. Valproic acid
D. Lamotrigine

Q214. Which of these medications is an inhaled corticosteroid used for asthma maintenance?
A. Salmeterol
B. Albuterol
C. Fluticasone
D. Montelukast

Q215. Which of the following is a cholinesterase inhibitor used in Alzheimer's disease?
A. Donepezil
B. Memantine
C. Rivastigmine
D. Galantamine

Q216. Which of these medications is a calcium channel blocker used for angina?
A. Metoprolol
B. Amlodipine
C. Lisinopril
D. Furosemide

Q217. Which of the following medications is a corticosteroid used orally for inflammation?
A. Hydrocortisone
B. Prednisone
C. Dexamethasone
D. Triamcinolone

Q218. Which of these medications is a short-acting benzodiazepine for anxiety?
A. Diazepam
B. Clonazepam
C. Lorazepam
D. Alprazolam

Q219. Which medication is an HMG-CoA reductase inhibitor used to lower LDL cholesterol?
A. Simvastatin
B. Ezetimibe
C. Gemfibrozil

D. Niacin

Q220. Which of these drugs is an opioid analgesic with antitussive properties?

A. Hydromorphone
B. Codeine
C. Tramadol
D. Oxycodone

Q221. Which of the following antibiotics is known for causing "Red Man Syndrome" if infused too quickly?

A. Ceftriaxone
B. Vancomycin
C. Gentamicin
D. Azithromycin

Q222. Which drug is a nonsteroidal anti-inflammatory medication used to close a patent ductus arteriosus in neonates?

A. Naproxen
B. Ibuprofen
C. Indomethacin
D. Ketorolac

Q223. Which DEA form must a pharmacy use when ordering Schedule II controlled substances?

A. DEA Form 222
B. DEA Form 41
C. DEA Form 106
D. DEA Form 224

Q224. The Controlled Substances Act is enforced primarily by which federal agency?

A. FDA
B. DEA
C. CDC
D. OSHA

Q225. Schedule II medications may be refilled:

A. Unlimited times within 6 months
B. Five times within 6 months
C. Once only with pharmacist authorization
D. Not at all

Q226. Which DEA form must be completed when a controlled substance is stolen or lost?

A. DEA Form 41
B. DEA Form 222
C. DEA Form 106
D. DEA Form 363

Q227. How often must a complete controlled substance inventory be conducted under federal law?

A. Monthly
B. Quarterly
C. Annually
D. Every 2 years

Q228. Which act mandates tracking and tracing of prescription drugs throughout the supply chain?

A. Kefauver-Harris Amendment
B. Food and Drug Act of 1906
C. Drug Supply Chain Security Act (DSCSA)
D. Pure Food and Cosmetic Act

Q229. DEA Form 41 is used primarily to:
A. Register a pharmacy
B. Order controlled substances
C. Report the destruction of controlled drugs
D. Transfer Schedule II drugs to another pharmacy
Q230. Which controlled substance schedule has no accepted medical use and highest abuse potential?
A. Schedule I
B. Schedule II
C. Schedule III
D. Schedule IV
Q231. Which DEA number prefix indicates a mid-level practitioner such as a nurse practitioner or physician assistant?
A. A or B
B. M
C. X
D. F
Q232. How long must DEA Form 222 records be retained by a pharmacy?
A. 6 months
B. 1 year
C. 2 years
D. 5 years
Q233. What type of controlled substance record must be kept separately from other pharmacy records?
A. Schedule III–V invoices
B. Schedule II records
C. OTC purchases
D. Medication guides
Q234. Which DEA form is used by a pharmacy to initially register for controlled substance handling?
A. DEA Form 106
B. DEA Form 224
C. DEA Form 363
D. DEA Form 222
Q235. A pharmacy must notify the DEA within what time frame after discovering a significant controlled substance loss?
A. Immediately upon discovery
B. Within 24 hours
C. Within 72 hours
D. Within 7 days
Q236. Pseudoephedrine sales are regulated under which law?
A. Combat Methamphetamine Epidemic Act of 2005
B. DSCSA of 2013
C. Orphan Drug Act
D. Pure Food and Drug Act
Q237. Controlled substance prescriptions must include all the following except:
A. Prescriber's DEA number
B. Patient name and address
C. Pharmacy DEA number
D. Drug strength and quantity

Q238. Which schedule includes medications such as alprazolam and diazepam?
A. Schedule II
B. Schedule III
C. Schedule IV
D. Schedule V
Q239. The FDA uses which classification to indicate a drug recall that may cause serious health consequences or death?
A. Class I
B. Class II
C. Class III
D. Market Withdrawal
Q240. Which agency enforces the Drug Supply Chain Security Act?
A. DEA
B. FDA
C. CDC
D. EPA
Q241. Controlled substances must be stored:
A. On open shelves for easy access
B. In a secure, locked cabinet or dispersed through stock to prevent theft
C. In the same drawer as OTC medications
D. In the pharmacist's office
Q242. Which organization manages Risk Evaluation and Mitigation Strategies (REMS)?
A. DEA
B. FDA
C. CDC
D. Joint Commission
Q243. The DEA registration for a pharmacy must be renewed every:
A. 6 months
B. 1 year
C. 2 years
D. 3 years
Q244. Which DEA form is used to request authorization to destroy expired controlled substances on-site?
A. DEA Form 222
B. DEA Form 41
C. DEA Form 106
D. DEA Form 224
Q245. Under federal law, controlled substance records must be readily retrievable within:
A. 24 hours of request
B. 48 hours of request
C. 72 hours of request
D. 7 days of request
Q246. Which DEA form allows the transfer of Schedule I and II substances between registrants?
A. DEA Form 222
B. DEA Form 106
C. DEA Form 363
D. DEA Form 224a
Q247. How many controlled substance schedules exist under the Controlled Substances Act?

A. 3
B. 4
C. 5
D. 6

Q248. What is the maximum quantity of pseudoephedrine a consumer may purchase per day under federal law?
A. 2.4 grams
B. 3.6 grams
C. 6 grams
D. 9 grams

Q249. What schedule includes cough syrups containing codeine?
A. Schedule II
B. Schedule III
C. Schedule IV
D. Schedule V

Q250. Which agency regulates the disposal of hazardous pharmaceutical waste?
A. EPA
B. DEA
C. FDA
D. CDC

Q251. Which of the following is a Schedule III drug?
A. Morphine
B. Hydrocodone/acetaminophen
C. Anabolic steroids
D. Alprazolam

Q252. The Food, Drug, and Cosmetic Act of 1938 was created to ensure:
A. Medication efficacy
B. Drug safety before marketing
C. Controlled substance regulation
D. Tracking of distribution

Q253. What information must appear on a controlled substance prescription label?
A. Prescriber's DEA number
B. Pharmacy DEA number
C. "Caution: Federal law prohibits the transfer..." statement
D. Pharmacist initials only

Q254. DEA Form 363 is required for:
A. Narcotic treatment programs
B. Hospital pharmacy registration
C. Ordering Schedule II drugs
D. Reporting destruction of controlled substances

Q255. Schedule III and IV prescriptions may be refilled up to:
A. 3 times in 3 months
B. 5 times in 6 months
C. 10 times in 12 months
D. Unlimited times with authorization

Q256. Which federal law first established five schedules for controlled substances?
A. Controlled Substances Act of 1970
B. Food, Drug, and Cosmetic Act

C. Drug Listing Act of 1972
D. Durham-Humphrey Amendment
Q257. Controlled substances must be inventoried:
A. Only for Schedule II drugs
B. When requested by the FDA
C. On the date the pharmacy first opens
D. Only after DEA inspection
Q263. Which schedule includes pregabalin (Lyrica)?
A. Schedule II
B. Schedule III
C. Schedule IV
D. Schedule V
Q264. Which organization regulates the labeling and advertising of prescription drugs?
A. FTC
B. DEA
C. FDA
D. CDC
Q265. A DEA Form 222 consists of how many copies?
A. One
B. Two
C. Three
D. Four
Q266. Which of the following is NOT required on a DEA Form 222?
A. Name of controlled substance
B. Supplier's name and address
C. DEA number of supplier
D. Patient's name and address
Q267. The federal agency responsible for classifying controlled substances into schedules is the:
A. FDA
B. DEA
C. CDC
D. EPA
Q268. The Kefauver-Harris Amendment of 1962 required manufacturers to prove:
A. Drug safety only
B. Drug safety and effectiveness
C. Labeling compliance
D. DEA registration
Q269. How long must pharmacies keep controlled substance inventories on file?
A. 6 months
B. 1 year
C. 2 years
D. 5 years
Q270. Which of the following drugs requires a DEA Form 222 for ordering?
A. Diazepam
B. Codeine-guaifenesin syrup
C. Methylphenidate
D. Tramadol
Q271. What is the maximum number of refills permitted for a Schedule III prescription?

A. 2
B. 3
C. 5
D. Unlimited

Q272. Which of the following describes a Schedule IV controlled substance?
A. No accepted medical use
B. Moderate abuse potential
C. High abuse potential
D. Low abuse potential relative to Schedule III

Q273. Which act distinguished between prescription and nonprescription drugs?
A. Controlled Substances Act
B. Durham-Humphrey Amendment
C. Kefauver-Harris Amendment
D. DSCSA

Q274. How soon must controlled-substance theft be reported to local police and the DEA?
A. Within 24 hours
B. Within 48 hours
C. Immediately upon discovery
D. Within 7 days

Q275. Which controlled-substance schedule includes Lomotil (diphenoxylate with atropine)?
A. Schedule II
B. Schedule III
C. Schedule IV
D. Schedule V

Q276. Which recordkeeping practice satisfies DEA requirements?
A. Combine all prescription records
B. Maintain Schedule II separately
C. Shred outdated forms monthly
D. Store records off-site without notice

Q277. How should controlled-substance prescriptions be filed if a pharmacy uses a three-file system?
A. Schedule II, Schedule III–V, and noncontrolled
B. Schedule I, Schedule II, and Schedule III–V
C. Schedule II–III, Schedule IV–V, and OTC
D. All controlled together, noncontrolled separate

Q278. What is the DEA number check formula used for validation?
A. (1+3+5)×1 + (2+4+6)×2
B. (1+3+5) + (2+4+6)×2, last digit matches seventh
C. Sum all digits equals 9
D. Multiply all odd digits by 2

Q279. A Class II FDA recall indicates:
A. Temporary health issues possible
B. Serious or fatal risk
C. Labeling violation only
D. No recall required

Q280. Which law created the DEA?
A. Controlled Substances Act
B. Drug Listing Act
C. Pure Food and Drug Act

D. DSCSA

Q281. Which label requirement is unique to controlled-substance prescriptions?

A. Pharmacy phone number
B. Federal transfer warning
C. Refill instructions
D. Prescriber signature

Q282. Which act authorized electronic prescribing of controlled substances (EPCS)?

A. HIPAA
B. DEA Interim Final Rule 2010
C. DSCSA 2013
D. Kefauver-Harris 1962

Q283. What is the purpose of the Risk Evaluation and Mitigation Strategies (REMS) program?

A. To classify controlled substances
B. To prevent counterfeiting in the drug supply chain
C. To ensure certain medications are used safely
D. To monitor over-the-counter drug advertising

Q284. Which of the following must be documented in the pseudoephedrine sales logbook?

A. Buyer's Social Security number
B. Buyer's name, address, and date/time of sale
C. Prescriber's DEA number
D. Manufacturer's lot number

Q285. Schedule II prescriptions must be stored for at least:

A. 6 months
B. 1 year
C. 2 years
D. 5 years

Q286. What is the federal limit on mail-order pseudoephedrine sales per 30 days?

A. 3.6 grams
B. 7.5 grams
C. 9 grams
D. 15 grams

Q287. Which act requires child-resistant packaging for most prescription medications?

A. Food, Drug, and Cosmetic Act
B. Poison Prevention Packaging Act
C. Controlled Substances Act
D. Drug Listing Act

Q288. When transferring a Schedule III–V prescription, the transferring pharmacist must document:

A. Only patient name and prescriber
B. DEA numbers of both pharmacies
C. Reason for transfer only
D. Insurance provider information

Q289. A DEA Form 222 order becomes invalid if:

A. It contains more than 10 items
B. The supplier's address changes
C. Any alteration or erasure is made
D. It is mailed without signature

Q290. Which organization manages the National Drug Code (NDC) system?

A. DEA

B. FDA
C. CDC
D. EPA

Q291. A pharmacy discovers an outdated Schedule II medication. What is the proper method for disposal?
A. Trash disposal
B. Flush down drain
C. Return to DEA-registered reverse distributor
D. Mail back to manufacturer directly

Q292. Which agency issues the NIOSH hazardous drug list used in pharmacy safety standards?
A. DEA
B. FDA
C. NIOSH (CDC)
D. EPA

Q293. Which controlled substance schedule includes buprenorphine?
A. Schedule II
B. Schedule III
C. Schedule IV
D. Schedule V

Q294. What is the main purpose of the Drug Enforcement Administration Number (DEA number)?
A. Identify prescribers authorized to prescribe controlled substances
B. Classify new drugs
C. Verify insurance coverage
D. Assign storage locations

Q295. The Controlled Substance Ordering System (CSOS) is used for:
A. Electronic ordering of Schedule II drugs
B. Electronic prescribing of noncontrolled drugs
C. Verifying patient refills
D. Reporting medication errors

Q296. Which type of recall involves a drug that is unlikely to cause adverse health effects but violates labeling requirements?
A. Class I
B. Class II
C. Class III
D. Market withdrawal

Q297. Under DEA regulations, which of the following actions requires a new registration?
A. Changing the pharmacy phone number
B. Relocating the pharmacy to a new address
C. Hiring new staff
D. Changing inventory software

Q298. Which of the following drugs is a Schedule IV controlled substance?
A. Codeine
B. Alprazolam
C. Hydrocodone
D. Methylphenidate

Q299. What must a pharmacist do before filling a controlled substance prescription from another state?
A. Verify prescriber DEA registration and state licensure

B. Automatically refuse to fill
C. Contact the DEA for approval
D. Report to FDA first

Q300. Which controlled substance schedule includes medications with accepted medical use but high abuse potential, such as oxycodone?

A. Schedule I
B. Schedule II
C. Schedule III
D. Schedule IV

Answer key and Explanation (201-300)

Q201. Answer: A

Explanation: Loratadine blocks H_1 receptors, relieving sneezing, itching, and runny nose without causing sedation. Dextromethorphan suppresses cough, guaifenesin loosens mucus, and montelukast reduces inflammation via leukotriene blockade. Loratadine is ideal for daily allergy management due to minimal drowsiness.

Q202. Answer: B

Explanation: Azithromycin and clarithromycin are macrolides that inhibit bacterial protein synthesis by binding the 50S ribosomal subunit. Cephalosporins affect cell walls, aminoglycosides target 30S ribosomes, and tetracyclines block tRNA attachment. Macrolides are effective for respiratory and soft tissue infections.

Q203. Answer: A

Explanation: Nitroglycerin releases nitric oxide, relaxing vascular smooth muscle and improving myocardial oxygen delivery. Furosemide is a diuretic, metoprolol a beta-blocker, and verapamil a calcium-channel blocker. Sublingual nitroglycerin acts within minutes but must be stored properly to preserve potency.

Q204. Answer: B

Explanation: Phenytoin causes gingival tissue overgrowth due to fibroblast stimulation, especially with poor dental hygiene. Valproic acid can cause hepatotoxicity, while levetiracetam and topiramate lack this effect. Patients should maintain oral hygiene and regular dental care during long-term use.

Q205. Answer: B

Explanation: Buspirone acts on serotonin receptors without sedation or dependence, making it ideal for chronic anxiety management. Alprazolam is for short-term anxiety, zolpidem for sleep, and hydroxyzine for acute anxiety. Buspirone's onset is delayed, requiring several weeks for full effect.

Q206. Answer: A

Explanation: Albuterol is a short-acting beta-2 agonist providing quick relief during asthma attacks. Fluticasone is preventive, montelukast controls inflammation, and salmeterol is long-acting for maintenance. Technicians should instruct patients to prime inhalers and monitor usage frequency.

Q207. Answer: B

Explanation: Bupropion inhibits dopamine and norepinephrine reuptake, reducing nicotine cravings and depressive symptoms. Paroxetine, fluoxetine, and sertraline are SSRIs without smoking cessation benefits. Patients should take it in the morning to minimize insomnia and report mood changes promptly.

Q208. Answer: B

Explanation: Lithium stabilizes mood in bipolar disorder but has a narrow therapeutic index, necessitating regular serum level monitoring. Risperidone, haloperidol, and quetiapine are antipsychotics. Dehydration or sodium imbalance increases lithium toxicity risk, requiring technician counseling on hydration.

Q209. Answer: B

Explanation: Lidocaine is a class IB antiarrhythmic that blocks sodium channels, stabilizing cardiac membranes and preventing ventricular arrhythmias. Amiodarone blocks potassium channels, digoxin increases contractility, and verapamil blocks calcium channels. Lidocaine is often used acutely via IV route.

Q210. Answer: C

Explanation: Famotidine reduces stomach acid by blocking histamine H_2 receptors on parietal cells. Omeprazole is a proton pump inhibitor, sucralfate protects ulcers, and misoprostol prevents NSAID-induced damage. Famotidine provides quick relief with fewer long-term risks than PPIs.

Q211. Answer: A
Explanation: Fluconazole inhibits fungal ergosterol synthesis and is effective for vulvovaginal candidiasis. Mupirocin targets bacteria, metronidazole treats anaerobic infections, and nystatin is for oral or cutaneous fungal infections. A single 150 mg oral dose is typically curative for most patients.
Q212. Answer: B
Explanation: Clozapine can cause severe neutropenia (agranulocytosis), requiring frequent CBC monitoring. Risperidone and olanzapine have metabolic side effects, while haloperidol carries EPS risk. Technicians must verify patient registration in REMS programs before dispensing clozapine.
Q213. Answer: B
Explanation: Gabapentin modulates calcium channels to reduce neuronal excitability, treating seizures and neuropathic pain. Phenytoin prevents generalized seizures, valproic acid affects GABA, and lamotrigine stabilizes sodium channels. Drowsiness and dizziness are common side effects that lessen with continued use.
Q214. Answer: C
Explanation: Fluticasone decreases airway inflammation and prevents asthma exacerbations. Salmeterol is a long-acting bronchodilator, albuterol offers rescue relief, and montelukast is oral adjunct therapy. Rinsing the mouth after use prevents oral thrush from local steroid deposition.
Q215. Answer: A
Explanation: Donepezil increases acetylcholine levels by inhibiting its breakdown, improving cognition in Alzheimer's disease. Memantine blocks NMDA receptors, while rivastigmine and galantamine are alternatives with shorter action. Donepezil is dosed once daily and well tolerated in mild to moderate dementia.
Q216. Answer: B
Explanation: Amlodipine relaxes vascular smooth muscle by blocking calcium influx, reducing angina and hypertension. Metoprolol is a beta-blocker, lisinopril an ACE inhibitor, and furosemide a diuretic. Amlodipine's slow onset minimizes reflex tachycardia compared to other vasodilators.
Q217. Answer: B
Explanation: Prednisone suppresses inflammation and immune responses in asthma, arthritis, and allergic conditions. Hydrocortisone is topical, dexamethasone is long-acting, and triamcinolone is medium-potency topical. Tapering doses prevents adrenal insufficiency after long-term corticosteroid use.
Q218. Answer: D
Explanation: Alprazolam acts quickly to relieve anxiety and panic symptoms but has a short duration, increasing dependence risk. Diazepam and clonazepam last longer, while lorazepam is intermediate. Controlled dispensing and gradual withdrawal are essential to avoid rebound anxiety.
Q219. Answer: A
Explanation: Simvastatin reduces hepatic cholesterol synthesis, lowering LDL and cardiovascular risk. Ezetimibe blocks absorption, gemfibrozil lowers triglycerides, and niacin raises HDL. Statin therapy requires liver enzyme monitoring and nighttime dosing for optimal cholesterol control.
Q220. Answer: B
Explanation: Codeine binds opioid receptors to relieve pain and suppress cough reflex. Hydromorphone and oxycodone are stronger analgesics, while tramadol also acts on serotonin and norepinephrine. Codeine-containing products require caution for pediatric use due to variable metabolism.
Q221. Answer: B
Explanation: Vancomycin causes histamine release when infused rapidly, resulting in flushing, rash, and hypotension known as "Red Man Syndrome." Ceftriaxone, gentamicin, and azithromycin do not cause this reaction. Infusing vancomycin slowly over at least 60 minutes prevents this adverse event.
Q222. Answer: C

Explanation: Indomethacin inhibits prostaglandin synthesis, promoting closure of the ductus arteriosus in premature infants. Ibuprofen can also be used, but indomethacin is the traditional choice. Naproxen and ketorolac are adult analgesics not approved for this neonatal indication.

Q223. Answer: A

Explanation: DEA Form 222 is required for all transfers or orders of Schedule II controlled substances, ensuring traceability and accountability between suppliers and registrants. Form 41 is used for destruction, 106 for theft/loss, and 224 for registration. Understanding proper form use prevents regulatory violations and supports compliance with the Controlled Substances Act.

Q224. Answer: B

Explanation: The DEA (Drug Enforcement Administration) enforces the Controlled Substances Act, regulating manufacturing, distribution, and dispensing of controlled drugs. The FDA monitors safety and labeling, CDC handles public health, and OSHA oversees workplace safety. DEA authority ensures proper scheduling, record keeping, and compliance inspections within pharmacies.

Q225. Answer: D

Explanation: Schedule II controlled substances cannot be refilled under federal law. Each new dispensing requires a separate written or electronic prescription from an authorized prescriber. Refills apply only to Schedules III and IV (within 6 months and five refills max). This restriction prevents misuse and diversion of high-risk drugs like oxycodone and morphine.

Q226. Answer: C

Explanation: DEA Form 106 documents theft or significant loss of controlled substances. It includes details on quantities, circumstances, and corrective actions. Form 41 is for destruction, 222 for ordering, and 363 for narcotic treatment registration. Reporting promptly to the DEA and local law enforcement helps prevent diversion and ensures federal compliance.

Q227. Answer: D

Explanation: A biennial (once every 2 years) inventory of all controlled substances is required by the DEA to verify accuracy and prevent diversion. Although some states require more frequent counts, the federal minimum remains biennial. Regular audits enhance accountability and accurate record keeping in pharmacy operations.

Q228. Answer: C

Explanation: The DSCSA establishes a national system for tracking and tracing prescription drugs to detect counterfeit and illegitimate products. It requires serialization, transaction records, and verification at each distribution step. The other acts addressed drug quality or safety but did not mandate supply-chain traceability.

Q229. Answer: C

Explanation: DEA Form 41 records the authorized destruction of expired or damaged controlled substances. It must include drug details, quantities, and witness verification. Form 224 registers pharmacies, 222 orders Schedule II drugs, and 106 reports thefts. Accurate destruction documentation prevents diversion and ensures compliance.

Q230. Answer: A

Explanation: Schedule I drugs (like heroin, LSD, and MDMA) have no accepted medical use in the United States and a high potential for abuse. They cannot be dispensed under any circumstance. Schedules II–V allow decreasing levels of medical use and abuse risk, affecting prescription and record-keeping requirements.

Q231. Answer: B

Explanation: DEA registration numbers beginning with "M" identify mid-level practitioners (e.g., NPs, PAs). Letters "A," "B," and "F" denote physicians or hospitals, while "X" is assigned for DATA-waivered buprenorphine prescribers. Recognizing prefix types aids technicians in validating prescription authenticity and regulatory compliance.

Q232. Answer: C
Explanation: DEA requires that all executed Form 222 records be retained for a minimum of two years for inspection and audit. This ensures traceability of Schedule II transactions. Some states may mandate longer retention. Accurate record maintenance is vital to avoid DEA citations and inventory discrepancies.
Q233. Answer: B
Explanation: Schedule II records must be maintained separately from Schedules III–V and non-controlled drug records. This facilitates rapid DEA inspection and reduces errors. Lower schedules may be stored together if readily retrievable. Proper segregation ensures compliance and efficient audit tracking.
Q234. Answer: B
Explanation: DEA Form 224 is the initial registration application for retail pharmacies, hospitals, and clinics to dispense controlled substances. Form 363 is for narcotic treatment programs, 106 for theft reporting, and 222 for Schedule II ordering. Registration validates legal authority to handle scheduled drugs.
Q235. Answer: A
Explanation: Federal law requires immediate notification to the DEA upon discovery of a significant loss or theft of controlled substances, followed by submission of Form 106. Prompt reporting protects public safety and demonstrates due diligence in diversion prevention.
Q236. Answer: A
Explanation: The Combat Methamphetamine Epidemic Act (2005) restricts the sale of pseudoephedrine-containing products, requiring ID verification, logbooks, and daily/monthly purchase limits. This reduces methamphetamine production. Other laws do not govern these precursor chemicals.
Q237. Answer: C
Explanation: A controlled substance prescription requires patient information, drug details, directions, and the prescriber's DEA number. The pharmacy's DEA number is not part of the prescription but appears on records. Ensuring complete and accurate prescriptions supports legal dispensing and traceability.
Q238. Answer: C
Explanation: Schedule IV drugs like benzodiazepines (alprazolam, diazepam) have a lower abuse potential than Schedules I–III and accepted medical uses. They can be refilled up to five times within six months. Proper scheduling knowledge prevents misclassification errors in dispensing and record keeping.
Q239. Answer: A
Explanation: A Class I recall involves products that pose a serious or life-threatening risk to health. Class II recalls address temporary reversible effects, and Class III recalls cover minor labeling issues. Pharmacy technicians must identify recall types to act quickly and protect patients.
Q240. Answer: B
Explanation: The FDA administers and enforces the Drug Supply Chain Security Act (DSCSA), which ensures product traceability and serialization to prevent counterfeits. The DEA focuses on controlled substances, while CDC and EPA cover health and environmental concerns. FDA oversight ensures integrity of the drug supply.
Q241. Answer: B
Explanation: Federal law requires that controlled substances be kept in a locked cabinet or securely dispersed throughout stock to deter theft and diversion. Accessibility must balance security with workflow. Open shelves or unsecured locations violate DEA standards and pose safety risks.
Q242. Answer: B
Explanation: The FDA manages REMS programs to ensure the benefits of certain drugs outweigh their risks by requiring special dispensing procedures, monitoring, and patient education. The DEA oversees

scheduling and controlled substance compliance. Technicians must adhere to REMS requirements when dispensing applicable medications.

Q243. Answer: D

Explanation: DEA registration for retail pharmacies and practitioners must be renewed every three years using Form 224a. This renewal ensures ongoing compliance and eligibility to handle controlled substances. Pharmacies must monitor expiration dates carefully to avoid lapses that can halt controlled drug dispensing or trigger penalties.

Q244. Answer: B

Explanation: DEA Form 41 must be submitted for approval before a pharmacy destroys controlled substances on-site. It documents the method, witnesses, and quantities destroyed. This ensures DEA oversight and prevents diversion. Destruction may also occur through reverse distributors who submit the form on behalf of pharmacies.

Q245. Answer: C

Explanation: Federal law requires pharmacies to produce controlled substance records within 72 hours of a DEA request. "Readily retrievable" means they can be separated and identified quickly. Efficient record organization demonstrates compliance and avoids citations during inspections or audits.

Q246. Answer: A

Explanation: DEA Form 222 is used for any transfer or exchange of Schedule I or II substances between DEA registrants, such as from a wholesaler to a pharmacy or between pharmacies. Each party must retain copies for at least two years, ensuring controlled tracking.

Q247. Answer: C

Explanation: The Controlled Substances Act establishes five schedules (I–V) categorized by medical use and abuse potential. Schedule I drugs have no accepted use, while Schedule V has the lowest abuse risk. Understanding these schedules is fundamental for correct dispensing, storage, and documentation procedures.

Q248. Answer: B

Explanation: The Combat Methamphetamine Epidemic Act limits pseudoephedrine sales to 3.6 grams per day and 9 grams per 30 days. These restrictions help prevent diversion into methamphetamine production. Pharmacies must maintain logbooks and verify customer identification before completing such transactions.

Q249. Answer: D

Explanation: Cough preparations with limited amounts of codeine, such as guaifenesin-codeine syrup, are classified as Schedule V drugs due to their lower abuse potential. They may be dispensed without a prescription in some states. Pharmacists must still ensure record keeping and proper labeling.

Q250. Answer: A

Explanation: The Environmental Protection Agency (EPA) enforces regulations for the disposal of hazardous pharmaceutical waste under the Resource Conservation and Recovery Act (RCRA). This ensures toxic substances are disposed of safely without environmental harm. The DEA handles controlled substance disposal specifically.

Q251. Answer: C

Explanation: Anabolic steroids, such as testosterone, are classified as Schedule III drugs due to moderate abuse potential and accepted medical use. Morphine and hydrocodone are Schedule II, while alprazolam is Schedule IV. Recognizing schedule differences is essential for accurate prescription handling and refilling limits.

Q252. Answer: B

Explanation: The FD&C Act of 1938 mandated drug safety testing before marketing, following the sulfanilamide tragedy. It gave the FDA authority over product safety and labeling. Efficacy requirements came later under the 1962 Kefauver-Harris Amendment. This act laid the foundation for modern drug regulation.

Q253. Answer: C

Explanation: Federal law requires Schedule II–IV prescription labels to bear the caution statement: "Caution: Federal law prohibits the transfer of this drug to any person other than the patient for whom it was prescribed." This warns against diversion and reinforces controlled use.

Q254. Answer: A

Explanation: DEA Form 363 is used to register narcotic treatment programs authorized to dispense or administer controlled substances for addiction treatment. It is distinct from Form 224 (for pharmacies) and Form 41 (for destruction). Proper registration ensures compliance with federal opioid treatment regulations.

Q255. Answer: B

Explanation: Federal law allows Schedule III and IV prescriptions to be refilled up to five times within six months from the issue date. After that, a new prescription is required. This limit balances legitimate medical use with the need to control abuse potential.

Q256. Answer: A

Explanation: The Controlled Substances Act of 1970 created five schedules and centralized control under the DEA. It unified federal drug laws to regulate manufacturing, distribution, and use. The other acts addressed labeling or prescription status but not controlled classification.

Q257. Answer: C

Explanation: A complete controlled substance inventory must be performed on the day a pharmacy first begins operations and every two years thereafter. This initial count establishes baseline accountability for all scheduled drugs handled under DEA registration.

Q263. Answer: D

Explanation: Pregabalin (Lyrica) is classified as a Schedule V controlled substance, meaning it has a low potential for abuse relative to Schedule IV drugs. It's prescribed for neuropathic pain and seizures. Schedule V drugs can often be refilled more easily but still require careful record keeping and monitoring for misuse.

Q264. Answer: C

Explanation: The Food and Drug Administration (FDA) oversees prescription drug labeling, packaging, and advertising to ensure safety and accuracy. The Federal Trade Commission (FTC) regulates over-the-counter drug advertising instead. Proper labeling prevents patient confusion, ensures dosing accuracy, and helps detect potential medication errors.

Q265. Answer: C

Explanation: DEA Form 222 includes three carbon copies: Copy 1 for the supplier, Copy 2 for the DEA, and Copy 3 retained by the purchaser (pharmacy). Each order line must specify drug name, strength, and quantity. Triplicate documentation maintains accountability for Schedule I and II controlled substance transfers.

Q266. Answer: D

Explanation: DEA Form 222 documents wholesale or inter-pharmacy transfers—not individual prescriptions—so patient information is not required. Instead, the form includes product, quantity, supplier, and purchaser data. Confusing prescription documentation with transfer forms can cause compliance violations during DEA audits or inspections.

Q267. Answer: B

Explanation: The Drug Enforcement Administration (DEA) classifies controlled substances based on medical use, abuse potential, and safety dependence. Scheduling decisions are coordinated with the Department of Health and Human Services and the FDA. Accurate scheduling guides prescribers and technicians in dispensing and storage requirements.

Q268. Answer: B
Explanation: The Kefauver-Harris Amendment mandated manufacturers to demonstrate both safety and effectiveness before marketing a drug. Prompted by the thalidomide tragedy, it strengthened FDA oversight of clinical trials and advertising. This amendment remains central to modern pharmaceutical regulation and pre-approval review.
Q269. Answer: C
Explanation: Federal law requires all controlled-substance inventories, whether initial or biennial, to be kept for at least two years and be readily retrievable for DEA review. Many states require longer retention. Proper record keeping demonstrates accountability and prevents diversion.
Q270. Answer: C
Explanation: Methylphenidate (Ritalin) is a Schedule II stimulant, requiring DEA Form 222 for ordering or transfer. Diazepam is Schedule IV, codeine-guaifenesin Schedule V, and tramadol Schedule IV. Schedule II inventory controls are strict due to high abuse potential and diversion risks.
Q271. Answer: C
Explanation: Schedule III and IV prescriptions may be refilled up to five times within six months after issuance. Any additional refills require a new prescription. This limit curbs abuse while ensuring patients maintain continuity of legitimate therapy under physician supervision.
Q272. Answer: D
Explanation: Schedule IV drugs, such as benzodiazepines, possess a lower abuse potential compared with Schedule III substances and have accepted medical uses. They may lead to limited psychological or physical dependence. Accurate schedule awareness ensures proper dispensing limits and storage security.
Q273. Answer: B
Explanation: The 1951 Durham-Humphrey Amendment legally defined prescription ("legend") and over-the-counter drugs, requiring the legend statement "Caution: Federal law prohibits dispensing without a prescription." This law clarified pharmacist roles and improved medication control.
Q274. Answer: C
Explanation: A significant loss or theft of controlled substances must be reported immediately upon discovery to the DEA and local law enforcement, followed by submission of DEA Form 106. Prompt reporting prevents diversion, supports investigations, and demonstrates compliance.
Q275. Answer: D
Explanation: Lomotil is a Schedule V medication because diphenoxylate, an opioid derivative, is present in limited quantity and combined with atropine to discourage abuse. It's used to treat diarrhea. Recognizing such low-dose narcotic combinations prevents misclassification errors.
Q276. Answer: B
Explanation: DEA regulations require Schedule II records to be maintained separately from all others. Schedules III–V may be stored together if readily retrievable. Separate filing simplifies audits and ensures compliance. Improper storage could result in DEA citations.
Q277. Answer: A
Explanation: In a three-file system, pharmacies file Schedule II prescriptions separately, Schedule III–V together, and noncontrolled prescriptions separately. This ensures fast retrieval during DEA inspections and avoids record misplacement, maintaining accountability.
Q278. Answer: B
Explanation: To verify a DEA number, add the 1st, 3rd, and 5th digits; then add twice the sum of the 2nd, 4th, and 6th digits. The right-most digit of this total must match the 7th digit of the DEA number. Validation prevents fraudulent prescriptions.
Q279. Answer: A

Explanation: A Class II recall is issued when exposure to a product may cause temporary or reversible adverse effects, or the likelihood of serious harm is remote. Pharmacists must promptly remove such products and notify patients if necessary.

Q280. Answer: A

Explanation: The Controlled Substances Act of 1970 established the Drug Enforcement Administration to consolidate drug enforcement and regulation under one federal agency. It replaced earlier fragmented systems and centralized responsibility for controlled-substance oversight.

Q281. Answer: B

Explanation: Controlled-substance labels for Schedules II–IV must state "Caution: Federal law prohibits the transfer of this drug ..." to deter diversion. This caution is not required for noncontrolled drugs. Accurate labeling ensures compliance and reinforces safe handling.

Q282. Answer: B

Explanation: The DEA's 2010 Interim Final Rule authorized Electronic Prescriptions for Controlled Substances (EPCS), establishing secure authentication and auditing requirements. This modernized prescribing, reduced forgery, and improved monitoring through electronic health systems.

Q283. Answer: C

Explanation: REMS is an FDA-required safety program for drugs with serious risks, ensuring benefits outweigh potential harm. It may include prescriber certification, patient consent, or restricted dispensing. Technicians help implement these safeguards by verifying documentation and providing medication guides.

Q284. Answer: B

Explanation: The Combat Methamphetamine Epidemic Act mandates that pseudoephedrine logbooks record the purchaser's name, address, product, quantity, and transaction time/date. This ensures traceability and compliance. ID verification is required before sale to prevent diversion for illicit methamphetamine production.

Q285. Answer: C

Explanation: DEA requires Schedule II prescription records to be retained for a minimum of two years and kept separate from other prescriptions. Some states extend retention up to five years. Consistent record storage ensures audit readiness and supports regulatory compliance.

Q286. Answer: B

Explanation: Under the Combat Methamphetamine Epidemic Act, customers purchasing pseudoephedrine via mail or online are limited to 7.5 grams within 30 days. Retail limits are 3.6 grams per day and 9 grams per 30 days. These controls help prevent precursor chemical diversion into illegal methamphetamine manufacturing.

Q287. Answer: B

Explanation: The Poison Prevention Packaging Act (PPPA) mandates child-resistant containers for most prescription and OTC medications to reduce accidental poisonings. Exceptions exist for certain patient requests or exempt medications. Pharmacy technicians ensure compliance by verifying appropriate packaging for each dispensed product.

Q288. Answer: B

Explanation: Federal law requires both pharmacies' DEA numbers, original prescription details, and transfer date be documented when transferring Schedule III–V prescriptions. This ensures tracking and prevents duplicate dispensing. Schedule II prescriptions may not be transferred because refills are prohibited.

Q289. Answer: C

Explanation: DEA Form 222 cannot contain alterations or erasures; any correction invalidates the entire form. A new form must be issued. This strict rule maintains document integrity and prevents potential tampering or diversion of Schedule II substances.

Q290. Answer: B

Explanation: The FDA administers the National Drug Code system, assigning unique identifiers for each manufacturer, product, and package size. This 10-digit number improves drug tracking, recall management, and error reduction. Technicians use NDCs to verify correct drug selection during dispensing.

Q291. Answer: C

Explanation: Expired Schedule II medications must be transferred to a DEA-registered reverse distributor for destruction. The distributor completes DEA Form 222 for the transfer and Form 41 for destruction. This ensures secure handling and proper documentation to prevent diversion.

Q292. Answer: C

Explanation: The National Institute for Occupational Safety and Health (NIOSH), part of the CDC, maintains the hazardous drug list that guides handling, storage, and PPE standards in pharmaciesывайте. Technicians must follow these guidelines to minimize exposure to toxic or carcinogenic agents.

Q293. Answer: B

Explanation: Buprenorphine is a Schedule III controlled substance, used for pain management and opioid dependence treatment under strict DEA oversight. Its lower abuse potential compared to full agonists like morphine justifies its Schedule III status, though diversion prevention remains essential.

Q294. Answer: A

Explanation: A DEA number uniquely identifies healthcare providers authorized to prescribe controlled substances. It's required on all controlled prescriptions for verification and accountability. This identifier enables pharmacists and technicians to confirm prescriber legitimacy and prevent fraudulent prescribing.

Q295. Answer: A

Explanation: CSOS allows DEA-registered entities to electronically order Schedule II controlled substances using digital certificates, replacing paper Form 222. It speeds processing, reduces errors, and provides secure record storage while maintaining compliance with federal regulations.

Q296. Answer: C

Explanation: A Class III recall is issued for products unlikely to cause harm but that violate FDA labeling or manufacturing standards. Pharmacists still remove affected stock to maintain compliance. Class I and II recalls involve higher risk levels.

Q297. Answer: B

Explanation: Moving a pharmacy to a new physical address requires a new DEA registration number specific to that location. Registrations are nontransferable and site-specific. The DEA must be notified in advance to maintain legal dispensing authority.

Q298. Answer: B

Explanation: Alprazolam (Xanax) is a Schedule IV benzodiazepine with lower abuse potential than Schedule II or III drugs. Hydrocodone and methylphenidate are Schedule II, while codeine may appear in Schedule II–V depending on formulation. Correct scheduling prevents dispensing violations.

Q299. Answer: A

Explanation: Pharmacists must verify that the prescriber holds a valid DEA registration and is licensed in their state of practice before filling out-of-state controlled prescriptions. This prevents fraud and ensures prescription legitimacy under federal and state law.

Q300. Answer: B

Explanation: Schedule II drugs, including oxycodone, have legitimate medical use but a high potential for abuse and dependence. They require new prescriptions for each fill, no refills allowed. Proper documentation and monitoring are vital to prevent misuse.

Questions (301-400)

Q301. Which act established the legal distinction between prescription and OTC drugs?

A. Durham-Humphrey Amendment
B. Controlled Substances Act
C. Food, Drug, and Cosmetic Act
D. Kefauver-Harris Amendment

Q302. Under federal law, how long must a pharmacy keep executed DEA Form 222s?

A. 6 months
B. 1 year
C. 2 years
D. 3 years

Q303. A pharmacy receives an official DEA Form 222 with missing information. What should it do?

A. Fill the order anyway
B. Add missing details and process
C. Void the form and return it to the purchaser
D. Submit to DEA for correction

Q304. Controlled substance inventories must record which of the following details?

A. Patient name and prescriber
B. Drug name, strength, dosage form, and quantity on hand
C. Supplier DEA number
D. Sales records

Q305. What is the maximum number of items that may be ordered per line on DEA Form 222?

A. 5
B. 10
C. 12
D. 20

Q306. Which controlled substance schedule is tramadol classified under?

A. Schedule II
B. Schedule III
C. Schedule IV
D. Schedule V

Q307. Which act requires manufacturers to register with the FDA and list all commercially distributed drugs?

A. Drug Listing Act of 1972
B. Controlled Substances Act of 1970
C. DSCSA of 2013
D. Orphan Drug Act of 1983

Q308. Which DEA form is used for a pharmacy to renew its registration?

A. Form 41
B. Form 222
C. Form 224a
D. Form 363

Q309. Schedule V medications differ from Schedule IV drugs because they:

A. Have higher abuse potential
B. Are often available without a prescription in some states
C. Cannot be refilled
D. Require DEA Form 222 for ordering

Q310. DEA Form 224 is used to:
A. Apply for pharmacy registration
B. Record destruction of drugs
C. Order Schedule II drugs
D. Report theft of controlled substances
Q311. What is the purpose of the DSCSA?
A. To prevent prescription errors
B. To track and trace drugs throughout the supply chain
C. To monitor controlled-substance diversion
D. To classify new medications
Q312. Which of the following must be reported to the DEA using Form 106?
A. Inventory discrepancies
B. Prescription errors
C. Theft or significant loss of controlled substances
D. Expired medication disposal
Q313. The Ryan Haight Online Pharmacy Consumer Protection Act regulates:
A. Importation of generic drugs
B. Online sales of controlled substances
C. Advertising of OTC medications
D. Pricing of brand-name drugs
Q314. Schedule II controlled substances must be stored:
A. In unlocked bins for quick access
B. In a secure, locked cabinet or safely dispersed through stock
C. Separately by manufacturer
D. In the pharmacist's office
Q315. A prescriber's DEA number with an "X" indicates:
A. A mid-level practitioner
B. A temporary registration
C. Authorization to prescribe buprenorphine for opioid addiction
D. Registration renewal in process
Q316. Which of the following is true regarding controlled substance prescription transmission?
A. Schedule II prescriptions may be faxed and filled immediately
B. Faxed Schedule II prescriptions require the original hard copy before dispensing
C. Schedule III–V may never be faxed
D. Controlled substances cannot be e-prescribed
Q317. What is the maximum number of lines available on each DEA Form 222?
A. 5
B. 10
C. 20
D. 25
Q318. Which act requires manufacturers to prove drug safety before marketing?
A. Durham-Humphrey Amendment
B. Food, Drug, and Cosmetic Act of 1938
C. Controlled Substances Act
D. Kefauver-Harris Amendment
Q319. Which document allows reverse distributors to destroy controlled substances on behalf of a pharmacy?
A. DEA Form 222

B. DEA Form 41
C. DEA Form 224a
D. DEA Form 363

Q320. Which law created a framework for drug tracking and verification to combat counterfeit medications?

A. Controlled Substances Act
B. Drug Supply Chain Security Act (DSCSA)
C. Drug Listing Act
D. Prescription Drug Marketing Act

Q321. Under federal law, a pharmacist may partially fill a Schedule II prescription if:

A. The prescriber authorizes it
B. The patient cannot afford the full quantity
C. The pharmacy is out of stock
D. The drug is not on formulary

Q322. Which of the following acts requires the use of tamper-resistant prescription pads for Medicaid prescriptions?

A. Combat Methamphetamine Epidemic Act
B. Medicaid Tamper-Resistant Prescription Act
C. Controlled Substances Act
D. DSCSA

Q323. How long must pseudoephedrine logbooks be retained by pharmacies?

A. 30 days
B. 6 months
C. 1 year
D. 2 years

Q324. A prescriber issues a controlled-substance prescription missing the DEA number. What should the technician do?

A. Fill it immediately
B. Add the number from memory
C. Alert the pharmacist to verify before filling
D. File it for later use

Q325. The federal law that established classification of drugs into Schedules I–V is the:

A. Controlled Substances Act
B. Durham-Humphrey Amendment
C. Kefauver-Harris Amendment
D. Poison Prevention Packaging Act

Q326. Which DEA form must a reverse distributor use when receiving Schedule II substances from a pharmacy?

A. DEA Form 41
B. DEA Form 222
C. DEA Form 106
D. DEA Form 224

Q327. A controlled-substance prescription missing the patient's address is:

A. Still valid under DEA rules
B. Invalid until corrected
C. Valid if verbal authorization given
D. Processed with pharmacist initials

Q328. What type of error requires completion of DEA Form 222 again?

A. Typographical
B. Wrong supplier address
C. Any erasure or correction
D. Incorrect date of shipment

Q329. How many controlled-substance schedules may appear on a single DEA Form 222?
A. One
B. Two
C. Three
D. Five

Q330. Which law required proof of drug effectiveness before marketing?
A. Kefauver-Harris Amendment
B. Durham-Humphrey Amendment
C. Controlled Substances Act
D. FD&C Act

Q331. Which DEA form is used to request a duplicate or replacement registration certificate?
A. DEA Form 223
B. DEA Form 224a
C. DEA Form 363
D. DEA Form 41

Q332. The federal agency responsible for enforcing hazardous-waste disposal laws for pharmaceuticals is:
A. DEA
B. EPA
C. FDA
D. CDC

Q333. A prescription for a controlled substance written by a veterinarian must include:
A. Pet name and owner's name
B. Owner's address only
C. Animal species only
D. Owner's phone number

Q334. Under DEA rules, controlled substances transferred between pharmacies must:
A. Be reported using DEA Form 106
B. Occur only with DEA registration at both locations
C. Require FDA authorization
D. Be reported to state boards only

Q335. A DEA registration certificate must be:
A. Filed off-site in storage
B. Displayed at the registered location
C. Mailed to the supplier annually
D. Held only by the pharmacist-in-charge

Q336. Which act was enacted to prevent counterfeit drugs from entering the U.S. market?
A. Kefauver-Harris Amendment
B. Prescription Drug Marketing Act (PDMA)
C. Controlled Substances Act
D. Orphan Drug Act

Q337. How long must a pharmacy maintain DEA registration records?
A. 1 year
B. 5 years

C. 3 years
D. 2 years
Q338. What is required to verify a prescriber's DEA number is legitimate?
A. Call the DEA directly
B. Use the DEA number validation formula
C. Check the prescriber's medical license
D. Request patient consent
Q339. A pharmacist should refuse to fill a controlled-substance prescription if:
A. The patient is new
B. The prescriber is from another state
C. The prescription appears forged or altered
D. The quantity is large
Q340. A DEA Form 106 should be filed when:
A. Drugs are expired
B. A controlled substance is stolen or lost
C. Drugs are transferred to another pharmacy
D. A pharmacist resigns
Q341. Which agency is responsible for enforcing laws related to controlled substance diversion and trafficking?
A. FDA
B. DEA
C. CDC
D. EPA
Q342. When must a pharmacy perform an initial controlled substance inventory?
A. Within the first year of operation
B. On the first day the pharmacy opens and handles controlled substances
C. After DEA inspection
D. After receiving first shipment
Q343. Which of the following best describes a Schedule III substance?
A. No medical use, high abuse potential
B. Moderate abuse potential and accepted medical use
C. Lowest abuse potential, OTC availability
D. High abuse potential and severe dependence risk
Q344. How often must controlled substance inventory be conducted under DEA regulations?
A. Every 6 months
B. Every year
C. Every 2 years
D. Every 5 years
Q345. A pharmacist discovers an outdated controlled drug. Which action complies with federal law?
A. Destroy it immediately
B. Return it to the manufacturer
C. Send it to a DEA-registered reverse distributor
D. Report to FDA first
Q346. Controlled substance prescriptions must include which information?
A. Pharmacy DEA number
B. Prescriber DEA number and signature
C. Patient insurance information
D. Supplier address

Q347. The main purpose of DEA Form 41 is to:
A. Register a new pharmacy
B. Record destruction of controlled substances
C. Report significant loss
D. Track pseudoephedrine sales
Q348. What is the penalty for a pharmacy that fails to maintain accurate controlled substance records?
A. License renewal delay
B. Civil fines or DEA registration revocation
C. Verbal warning only
D. Local citation
Q349. Which agency regulates the disposal of hazardous non-controlled pharmaceuticals?
A. DEA
B. FDA
C. EPA
D. CDC
Q350. Schedule II controlled substances include:
A. Acetaminophen with codeine
B. Alprazolam
C. Oxycodone
D. Lomotil
Q351. What is the main purpose of the Controlled Substance Ordering System (CSOS)?
A. To report lost controlled substances
B. To electronically order Schedule II substances
C. To destroy expired medications
D. To validate prescriber credentials
Q352. What is the primary difference between Schedule I and Schedule II drugs?
A. Schedule I drugs have no accepted medical use
B. Schedule I drugs can be refilled
C. Schedule II drugs have higher abuse potential
D. Schedule II drugs cannot be prescribed
Q353. The Combat Methamphetamine Epidemic Act requires what for pseudoephedrine purchases?
A. Pharmacist-only sales
B. Prescription for all products
C. Photo ID and logbook entry
D. DEA form submission
Q354. What type of DEA registration is required for a hospital pharmacy?
A. Form 363
B. Form 224
C. Form 41
D. Form 106
Q355. Which class of recall is issued when a product could cause temporary or reversible adverse effects?
A. Class I
B. Class II
C. Class III
D. Market withdrawal
Q356. Which DEA form is required for reporting the destruction of expired controlled substances?
A. DEA Form 222

B. DEA Form 224
C. DEA Form 106
D. DEA Form 41

Q357. Which act established penalties for unauthorized distribution of controlled substances?
A. Food, Drug, and Cosmetic Act
B. Controlled Substances Act
C. Drug Listing Act
D. Durham-Humphrey Amendment

Q358. A DEA Form 224a is used to:
A. Apply for an initial DEA registration
B. Renew a DEA registration
C. Report drug theft or loss
D. Transfer controlled substances

Q359. What is required when transferring Schedule III–V controlled substances to another pharmacy?
A. DEA Form 222
B. Standard invoice documenting the transfer
C. DEA Form 41
D. DEA Form 106

Q360. What is the function of the DEA Diversion Control Division?
A. Approve new drug products
B. Oversee marketing of nonprescription drugs
C. Prevent, detect, and investigate controlled-substance diversion
D. Track controlled-substance imports only

Q361. What does the DSCSA require pharmacies to do with suspect or illegitimate drugs?
A. Destroy them immediately
B. Quarantine and investigate them
C. Dispense them with warning labels
D. Report only to manufacturers

Q362. A controlled substance inventory must include which of the following for Schedule II drugs?
A. Estimated count
B. Exact count
C. Volume-based measurement
D. Weight in milligrams

Q363. The FDA can issue which type of recall for a drug likely to cause death or serious harm?
A. Class I
B. Class II
C. Class III
D. Market withdrawal

Q364. The Combat Methamphetamine Epidemic Act restricts pseudoephedrine sales to no more than:
A. 2.4 grams daily and 6 grams monthly
B. 3.6 grams daily and 9 grams monthly
C. 4.5 grams daily and 12 grams monthly
D. 6 grams daily and 18 grams monthly

Q365. What is the DEA's authority for revoking a registration?
A. Lack of business license
B. Violation of Controlled Substances Act regulations
C. Employee turnover
D. Change in insurance provider

Q366. Which controlled substance schedule includes medications like Tylenol #3 (codeine with acetaminophen)?
A. Schedule II
B. Schedule III
C. Schedule IV
D. Schedule V
Q367. DEA Form 223 is used for:
A. Duplicate or replacement registration certificate
B. Schedule II ordering
C. Registration renewal
D. Theft reporting
Q368. Which organization publishes the list of hazardous drugs used in healthcare settings?
A. DEA
B. NIOSH
C. FDA
D. OSHA
Q369. What is the primary purpose of DEA Form 222?
A. To report drug theft
B. To order or transfer Schedule I or II drugs
C. To register new facilities
D. To document destruction of controlled substances
Q370. Which act gave the DEA the authority to regulate controlled substances?
A. Controlled Substances Act
B. Pure Food and Drug Act
C. Kefauver-Harris Amendment
D. Drug Listing Act
Q371. Which controlled substance schedule includes drugs like cough syrups with limited amounts of codeine?
A. Schedule II
B. Schedule III
C. Schedule IV
D. Schedule V
Q372. What document must a pharmacy maintain to prove controlled-substance disposal?
A. DEA Form 106
B. DEA Form 41
C. DEA Form 224
D. DEA Form 363
Q373. Which schedule includes drugs with the lowest abuse potential?
A. Schedule II
B. Schedule III
C. Schedule IV
D. Schedule V
Q374. Under federal law, pharmacies must report controlled-substance theft to:
A. DEA and local police
B. State board only
C. FDA and CDC
D. Manufacturer only
Q375. DEA-registered pharmacies must renew their registration every:

A. Year
B. Two years
C. Three years
D. Five years

Q376. Which of the following medications is classified as high-alert and requires verification by a second technician or pharmacist before dispensing?
A. Ibuprofen
B. Lisinopril
C. Insulin glargine
D. Loratadine

Q377. A pharmacy technician notices "hydralazine" and "hydroxyzine" stored next to each other on the shelf. What safety action should be taken?
A. Leave them as is
B. Apply Tall Man lettering and separate storage
C. Remove hydroxyzine from inventory
D. Re-label only hydralazine

Q378. Which type of error occurs when the wrong strength of the correct medication is dispensed?
A. Omission error
B. Wrong dose error
C. Wrong drug error
D. Wrong time error

Q379. When should a technician refer a patient to the pharmacist for counseling?
A. When a patient asks about drug interactions
B. When verifying refill eligibility
C. When printing medication labels
D. When counting tablets

Q380. What is the main purpose of a root-cause analysis (RCA) following a medication error?
A. Identify who made the mistake
B. Determine the underlying system failures
C. Report the pharmacist to the board
D. Record employee disciplinary actions

Q381. Which organization operates the MedWatch program?
A. CDC
B. FDA
C. ISMP
D. DEA

Q382. Which action best prevents cross-contamination when counting hazardous tablets such as chemotherapy agents?
A. Use the same counting tray after wiping
B. Wear gloves and use a designated tray
C. Count directly on the countertop
D. Pour tablets back into the stock bottle

Q383. A pharmacy uses bar-code verification at the filling station. This primarily helps reduce which type of error?
A. Communication error
B. Dispensing error
C. Prescribing error
D. Documentation error

Q384. The abbreviation "U" for "unit" should be avoided because it can be mistaken for:
A. Zero
B. Four
C. Ten
D. None of the above
Q385. Which procedure is most appropriate when a technician discovers a recalled medication on the shelf?
A. Discard it immediately in regular trash
B. Quarantine it and follow recall instructions
C. Continue using until official notice arrives
D. Return it to active inventory
Q386. A technician accidentally labels amoxicillin 500 mg as 250 mg. Which error category best describes this?
A. Labeling error
B. Wrong drug error
C. Omission error
D. Compliance error
Q387. Which infection-control practice must always precede handling sterile compounding supplies?
A. Cleaning counters with alcohol
B. Washing hands and forearms
C. Donning sterile gloves first
D. Spraying gloves with alcohol only
Q388. Which metric is typically used in Continuous Quality Improvement (CQI) programs to assess dispensing accuracy?
A. Customer satisfaction
B. Error rate per prescriptions filled
C. Prescription wait time
D. Technician payroll hours
Q389. What type of report should be filed for a near miss medication event?
A. No report is needed
B. Confidential quality-improvement report
C. Police report
D. Insurance claim
Q390. A patient experiences hives after taking amoxicillin. This reaction should be documented as:
A. Adverse drug event
B. Medication error
C. Noncompliance incident
D. Storage error
Q391. When a prescription appears to contain conflicting directions, the technician should:
A. Guess based on common dosing
B. Contact the pharmacist immediately
C. Call the prescriber directly
D. Ask another technician for advice
Q392. Which federal agency oversees enforcement of infection-control standards in the workplace?
A. FDA
B. OSHA
C. DEA
D. CDC

Q393. A technician observes another employee bypassing bar-code scanning to speed up workflow. What is the best immediate action?
A. Ignore it unless an error occurs
B. Report to the pharmacist or supervisor
C. Confront the coworker publicly
D. Shut down the workstation
Q394. Which of the following medications is look-alike/sound-alike with "Celebrex"?
A. Celexa
B. Cipro
C. Ceftin
D. Cephalexin
Q395. Which of the following is the most effective method for preventing medication-error recurrence?
A. Punishing the responsible employee
B. Conducting regular CQI meetings
C. Limiting staffing hours
D. Increasing prescription quotas
Q396. Which abbreviation is considered error-prone and should not be used on medication labels?
A. BID
B. QD
C. PO
D. PRN
Q397. Which type of error is prevented by using a bar-code administration system in hospitals?
A. Prescribing errors
B. Administration errors
C. Manufacturing errors
D. Procurement errors
Q398. A pharmacy technician notes an expired medication in the active stock area. What is the correct action?
A. Leave it for the next shift
B. Relabel with a new expiration date
C. Remove and quarantine for disposal
D. Mix it with new stock
Q399. Which organization issues recommendations for preventing medication errors and promotes the use of Tall Man lettering?
A. DEA
B. ISMP
C. CDC
D. OSHA
Q400. If a patient experiences nausea and vomiting after taking a medication correctly, what should this be classified as?
A. Prescribing error
B. Adverse drug reaction
C. Dispensing error
D. Administration error

Answer key and Explanation (301-400)

Q301. Answer: A

Explanation: The Durham-Humphrey Amendment (1951) defined prescription-only medications and required "Rx only" labeling. It also authorized verbal prescriptions and refills. This distinction guides pharmacists in dispensing and counseling responsibilities.

Q302. Answer: C

Explanation: DEA requires that executed Form 222s be retained for at least two years, readily retrievable for audit. These forms document every Schedule II transaction, supporting inventory accuracy and preventing diversion.

Q303. Answer: C

Explanation: Any DEA Form 222 that contains incomplete or incorrect information must be voided and returned to the purchaser. Altering the form invalidates it under federal law. This ensures accurate documentation and prevents diversion of Schedule II controlled substances.

Q304. Answer: B

Explanation: A controlled substance inventory must include each drug's name, strength, dosage form, and quantity on hand. This baseline data allows DEA inspectors to verify stock levels and detect discrepancies. Patient or sales information is not part of inventory documentation.

Q305. Answer: B

Explanation: Each DEA Form 222 allows up to 10 line items for ordering Schedule I or II controlled substances. Each line corresponds to a separate drug name and strength. The form's structure ensures standardized ordering and traceability between supplier and purchaser.

Q306. Answer: C

Explanation: Tramadol is classified as a Schedule IV controlled substance due to its moderate abuse potential compared with Schedule II opioids. It's used for pain management and must be dispensed following DEA regulations on refills and labeling.

Q307. Answer: A

Explanation: The Drug Listing Act of 1972 requires all drug manufacturers, packagers, and distributors to register with the FDA and provide detailed product lists. This law also established the National Drug Code (NDC) system used for drug identification.

Q308. Answer: C

Explanation: DEA Form 224a is used to renew a pharmacy's controlled substance registration every three years. Renewal maintains authorization to handle controlled substances legally. Using outdated registration can result in DEA penalties or suspension.

Q309. Answer: B

Explanation: Schedule V drugs, such as certain cough syrups with codeine, have the lowest abuse potential and may be available OTC in some states. They do not require DEA Form 222 and can be refilled more freely than higher schedules.

Q310. Answer: A

Explanation: DEA Form 224 is the application for initial registration of pharmacies, hospitals, or clinics to dispense controlled substances. Without an approved 224 registration, facilities cannot legally handle scheduled drugs.

Q311. Answer: B

Explanation: The Drug Supply Chain Security Act (DSCSA) establishes a national system for tracking prescription drugs from manufacturer to dispenser. It ensures product legitimacy, prevents counterfeit distribution, and mandates serialization and transaction data.

Q312. Answer: C

Explanation: DEA Form 106 reports theft or significant loss of controlled substances. Pharmacies must file this form immediately upon discovery and notify local law enforcement. This ensures accountability and assists investigations into potential diversion incidents.

Q313. Answer: B

Explanation: The Ryan Haight Act restricts online pharmacies from dispensing controlled substances without valid prescriptions issued after at least one in-person medical evaluation. It combats illegal Internet drug sales and ensures patient safety.

Q314. Answer: B

Explanation: DEA regulations require Schedule II drugs to be securely stored in a locked cabinet or dispersed among other inventory to prevent theft. This dual option ensures safety while maintaining efficient workflow.

Q315. Answer: C

Explanation: A DEA number beginning with "X" designates a DATA-waivered prescriber authorized to prescribe buprenorphine for opioid-use disorder treatment. This supports controlled, monitored addiction therapy under the Drug Addiction Treatment Act.

Q316. Answer: B

Explanation: Schedule II prescriptions sent by fax require the original signed hard copy before dispensing unless for long-term care, hospice, or parenteral administration. Schedule III–V may be faxed or e-prescribed directly. This ensures authenticity and prevents fraudulent orders for high-risk drugs.

Q317. Answer: B

Explanation: Each DEA Form 222 contains ten lines, each for a separate Schedule I or II drug. Using the form correctly ensures complete documentation and regulatory compliance during transfers between registered entities. Altered or incomplete forms are invalid under DEA rules.

Q318. Answer: B

Explanation: The Food, Drug, and Cosmetic Act of 1938 mandated safety testing for all new drugs after the sulfanilamide disaster. It granted the FDA authority to review applications before marketing. Later amendments expanded requirements to include proof of efficacy and labeling standards.

Q319. Answer: B

Explanation: DEA Form 41 documents the destruction of controlled substances, whether performed by the pharmacy or an authorized reverse distributor. This ensures accountability and compliance with federal laws requiring witnessed destruction to prevent diversion.

Q320. Answer: B

Explanation: The 2013 DSCSA established nationwide drug tracking, verification, and serialization standards to prevent counterfeit or diverted drugs from entering the U.S. supply chain. It requires pharmacies to maintain transaction documentation for six years.

Q321. Answer: C

Explanation: Federal law permits partial filling of Schedule II prescriptions if the pharmacy has insufficient stock, provided the remainder is supplied within 72 hours. Partial fills are also allowed for terminally ill or LTCF patients under different timelines.

Q322. Answer: B

Explanation: The Medicaid Tamper-Resistant Prescription Act mandates that all written Medicaid prescriptions be issued on tamper-resistant pads to prevent forgery or unauthorized copying. This measure significantly reduces prescription fraud and diversion.

Q323. Answer: D

Explanation: Pharmacies must retain pseudoephedrine sales logbooks for at least two years under the Combat Methamphetamine Epidemic Act. These records must be accessible for law enforcement review to verify compliance and detect suspicious purchasing patterns.

Q324. Answer: C

Explanation: Controlled-substance prescriptions missing a DEA number cannot be filled until verified by the pharmacist. The DEA number confirms prescriber authorization. Unauthorized filling could result in severe regulatory penalties or diversion risks.

Q325. Answer: A

Explanation: The Controlled Substances Act of 1970 created five drug schedules and consolidated federal drug laws. It remains the foundation of controlled-substance regulation, enforced by the DEA to control manufacture, distribution, and dispensing.

Q326. Answer: B

Explanation: Reverse distributors must complete DEA Form 222 to receive Schedule II substances from a pharmacy. This form documents the transfer for accountability and ensures proper handling prior to destruction.

Q327. Answer: B

Explanation: Federal law requires patient name, address, and prescriber DEA number on every controlled-substance prescription. Missing information renders it invalid until corrected by the prescriber. This ensures accurate identification and prevents fraudulent use.

Q328. Answer: C

Explanation: Any erasure, strikeout, or correction on DEA Form 222 invalidates it entirely. A new form must be completed to ensure authenticity. Maintaining unaltered documentation is key to preventing compliance issues during audits.

Q329. Answer: A

Explanation: DEA Form 222 can only include substances from a single schedule—Schedule I or II. Combining multiple schedules on the same form violates DEA regulations and invalidates the order.

Q330. Answer: A

Explanation: The Kefauver-Harris Amendment of 1962 required evidence of both safety and efficacy before drug approval, following the thalidomide tragedy. It also established Good Manufacturing Practices (GMP) and informed consent standards for clinical trials.

Q331. Answer: A

Explanation: DEA Form 223 allows registrants to obtain a duplicate or replacement certificate if the original is lost or destroyed. Maintaining an updated registration on file ensures continuous authorization to handle controlled substances legally.

Q332. Answer: B

Explanation: The Environmental Protection Agency (EPA) enforces pharmaceutical hazardous waste disposal standards under the Resource Conservation and Recovery Act (RCRA). This prevents environmental contamination from toxic or reactive chemical disposal.

Q333. Answer: A

Explanation: Veterinary prescriptions for controlled substances must list both the animal's name and the owner's name and address to ensure traceability. This information identifies the end user and supports DEA compliance requirements.

Q334. Answer: B

Explanation: Both pharmacies must hold active DEA registrations to transfer controlled substances legally. Schedule II transfers require Form 222, while lower schedules use invoices. These records maintain compliance and tracking integrity.

Q335. Answer: B

Explanation: DEA registration certificates must be displayed prominently at the registered business location. This allows inspectors to confirm compliance during audits and demonstrates legal authorization for handling controlled substances.

Q336. Answer: B

Explanation: The Prescription Drug Marketing Act (PDMA) of 1987 was designed to prevent counterfeit, adulterated, or misbranded drugs from entering the supply chain. It regulates the distribution of drug samples and prohibits the re-importation of prescription medications to protect patients and maintain supply integrity.

Q337. Answer: D

Explanation: All DEA registration records must be kept for at least two years and be readily retrievable for inspection. This includes Form 224, renewals, and related documentation. Accurate record retention demonstrates ongoing compliance and ensures traceability during DEA audits.

Q338. Answer: B

Explanation: DEA numbers can be validated using the 7-digit formula: add the 1st, 3rd, and 5th digits to twice the sum of the 2nd, 4th, and 6th digits. The rightmost digit of that total should match the 7th digit. This check confirms legitimacy.

Q339. Answer: C

Explanation: Any controlled-substance prescription showing signs of forgery, alteration, or irregularities must be refused. Pharmacists should contact the prescriber and authorities if needed. Dispensing fraudulent prescriptions violates federal law and can result in DEA penalties.

Q340. Answer: B

Explanation: DEA Form 106 is required to document theft or significant loss of controlled substances. The pharmacy must notify the DEA and local authorities immediately upon discovery, then submit the completed form. Accurate reporting prevents diversion and ensures compliance with the Controlled Substances Act.

Q341. Answer: B

Explanation: The Drug Enforcement Administration (DEA) enforces federal laws related to controlled substances, including diversion prevention, trafficking investigations, and prescription regulation. The DEA's authority ensures safe handling, monitoring, and legal accountability within the pharmaceutical supply chain.

Q342. Answer: B

Explanation: Federal law requires an initial controlled substance inventory on the first day the pharmacy handles any controlled drugs. This establishes a baseline count for future biennial inventories, ensuring accurate recordkeeping and preventing discrepancies or diversion.

Q343. Answer: B

Explanation: Schedule III drugs, such as anabolic steroids and certain codeine combinations, have accepted medical uses and moderate abuse potential. They can cause low-to-moderate physical dependence or high psychological dependence, requiring controlled prescribing and refill limits.

Q344. Answer: C

Explanation: DEA regulations mandate a complete controlled substance inventory at least once every two years (biennially). The count must include all controlled drugs on hand. Some states may require more frequent inventories for tighter oversight.

Q345. Answer: C

Explanation: Expired or damaged controlled substances must be sent to a DEA-registered reverse distributor for proper disposal. The reverse distributor handles DEA Form 222 for Schedule II transfers and Form 41 for destruction. This process prevents diversion.

Q346. Answer: B

Explanation: Controlled substance prescriptions must contain the prescriber's DEA number, signature, patient name and address, drug name, strength, quantity, and directions. Missing or incomplete data makes the prescription invalid and illegal to fill under DEA rules.

Q347. Answer: B

Explanation: DEA Form 41 documents the destruction of expired or damaged controlled substances, including details about the drug, quantity, and method used. Witness verification ensures proper disposal under federal supervision, preventing diversion or misuse.

Q348. Answer: B

Explanation: Failure to maintain accurate controlled substance records can result in DEA fines, registration suspension, or criminal prosecution. Recordkeeping integrity is a cornerstone of compliance with the Controlled Substances Act.

Q349. Answer: C

Explanation: The Environmental Protection Agency (EPA) regulates hazardous waste disposal, including non-controlled pharmaceuticals under the Resource Conservation and Recovery Act (RCRA). This ensures drugs are disposed of in an environmentally safe manner, protecting water and soil quality.

Q350. Answer: C

Explanation: Oxycodone is a Schedule II opioid with high abuse potential but accepted medical use. These drugs require new prescriptions for each dispensing and cannot be refilled. Schedule III–V substances have lower abuse risks and may allow limited refills.

Q351. Answer: B

Explanation: CSOS enables DEA-registered entities to electronically order Schedule II controlled substances securely, replacing the paper Form 222. It streamlines transactions, reduces paperwork, and maintains full audit traceability under federal guidelines.

Q352. Answer: A

Explanation: Schedule I drugs, such as heroin or LSD, have no accepted medical use and are illegal for prescribing in the U.S. Schedule II drugs, like morphine or oxycodone, have medical use but strict control requirements.

Q353. Answer: C

Explanation: Consumers must present valid photo identification, and sales must be logged with date, purchaser details, and quantity under the Combat Methamphetamine Epidemic Act. This helps track transactions and prevent precursor misuse in methamphetamine manufacturing.

Q354. Answer: B

Explanation: Hospitals and retail pharmacies must file DEA Form 224 to obtain registration for handling controlled substances. This form establishes their authority to dispense and maintain compliance with DEA regulations.

Q355. Answer: B

Explanation: A Class II recall involves drugs that may cause temporary or reversible health effects, with a low probability of serious harm. Pharmacists must promptly remove affected stock and notify patients when applicable.

Q356. Answer: D

Explanation: DEA Form 41 is used to document the destruction of controlled substances. Pharmacies must submit it before disposal, detailing quantities and witnesses. This ensures secure, supervised destruction and prevents potential diversion or misuse of expired controlled medications.

Q357. Answer: B

Explanation: The Controlled Substances Act (CSA) of 1970 established legal penalties for unauthorized possession, distribution, or manufacture of controlled substances. It consolidated drug laws under the DEA to regulate scheduling, enforcement, and recordkeeping.

Q358. Answer: B

Explanation: DEA Form 224a renews a pharmacy's DEA registration every three years. This renewal maintains the facility's legal authority to dispense controlled substances. Failure to renew before expiration suspends controlled-substance handling privileges.

Q359. Answer: B

Explanation: Transfers of Schedule III–V drugs require an invoice documenting drug names, quantities, dates, and DEA numbers of both parties. DEA Form 222 is reserved for Schedule II transfers. Proper documentation prevents diversion and ensures accountability during inspections.

Q360. Answer: C

Explanation: The DEA Diversion Control Division monitors and enforces regulations to prevent the misuse and diversion of controlled substances into illicit channels. It conducts audits, investigations, and outreach to maintain compliance among registrants and healthcare professionals.

Q361. Answer: B

Explanation: The Drug Supply Chain Security Act mandates pharmacies quarantine and investigate suspect or illegitimate drugs. If confirmed, they must notify the FDA and trading partners within 24 hours. This system helps protect patients from counterfeit or adulterated products.

Q362. Answer: B

Explanation: Federal law requires an exact count of all Schedule II drugs during inventories. Estimated counts are only acceptable for Schedule III–V if containers hold ≤1000 units. Exact counting prevents discrepancies and diversion.

Q363. Answer: A

Explanation: A Class I recall is the most severe, reserved for drugs posing a reasonable probability of serious adverse health effects or death. Immediate removal from shelves and patient notification are required to prevent harm.

Q364. Answer: B

Explanation: The Combat Methamphetamine Epidemic Act limits retail pseudoephedrine sales to 3.6 grams per day and 9 grams per 30 days. These limits help prevent illegal synthesis of methamphetamine from common decongestant products.

Q365. Answer: B

Explanation: The DEA may revoke a registration if the registrant violates Controlled Substances Act rules, including poor recordkeeping, diversion, or fraudulent activity. Revocation halts legal handling of controlled substances and may result in prosecution.

Q366. Answer: B

Explanation: Codeine combinations containing ≤90 mg per dose unit, such as Tylenol #3, are classified as Schedule III drugs. They have moderate abuse potential and accepted medical use, subject to refill and prescription regulations.

Q367. Answer: A

Explanation: DEA Form 223 provides a duplicate copy of a lost or destroyed DEA registration certificate. It ensures registrants maintain proof of authorization to handle controlled substances during inspections or audits.

Q368. Answer: B

Explanation: The National Institute for Occupational Safety and Health (NIOSH) publishes and updates the hazardous drugs list, guiding safe handling, PPE use, and compounding procedures in healthcare facilities. This protects workers from exposure risks.

Q369. Answer: B

Explanation: DEA Form 222 is used to order or transfer Schedule I and II drugs between DEA-registered entities. It ensures accountability and traceability for high-risk controlled substances throughout the supply chain.

Q370. Answer: A

Explanation: The Controlled Substances Act of 1970 empowered the DEA to enforce drug control laws, establish schedules, and oversee manufacturing, distribution, and recordkeeping of controlled substances. It remains the cornerstone of U.S. drug regulation.

Q371. Answer: D

Explanation: Schedule V drugs have the lowest abuse potential and include cough syrups with limited codeine. They can sometimes be sold without a prescription depending on state law, but recordkeeping is still required.

Q372. Answer: B

Explanation: DEA Form 41 serves as official proof of controlled-substance destruction, documenting the drug name, strength, quantity, and destruction method. It must be witnessed and kept for at least two years for compliance review.

Q373. Answer: D

Explanation: Schedule V drugs, such as pregabalin and cough medications with small codeine quantities, have the lowest potential for abuse. They often have accepted medical uses and may be available without prescriptions in some states.

Q374. Answer: A

Explanation: Significant loss or theft of controlled substances must be reported immediately to both the DEA and local law enforcement. Prompt reporting and submission of DEA Form 106 prevent diversion and support investigations.

Q375. Answer: C

Explanation: Pharmacies must renew DEA registration every three years using Form 224a. This ensures continued authorization to handle controlled substances legally. Operating without renewal violates federal law and may lead to penalties or suspension.

Q376. Answer: C

Explanation: High-alert drugs, such as insulin, anticoagulants, and chemotherapy agents, pose a higher risk of harm if used incorrectly. Double-checking insulin glargine before dispensing prevents dosing errors. Lisinopril and ibuprofen are not high-alert, and loratadine is generally over-the-counter, carrying minimal risk when used correctly.

Q377. Answer: B

Explanation: Look-alike/sound-alike (LASA) medications should be separated physically and labeled with Tall Man lettering to reduce selection errors. Removing one drug or simply re-labeling one is insufficient. Organized shelving and distinct labeling maintain medication accuracy and patient safety across the dispensing process.

Q378. Answer: B

Explanation: Dispensing the correct medication at an incorrect strength represents a wrong dose error. Omission refers to failure to administer, wrong drug means the incorrect medication, and wrong time involves incorrect scheduling. Recognizing error categories helps technicians report accurately and support continuous quality improvement (CQI) efforts.

Q379. Answer: A

Explanation: Any patient question involving interactions, side effects, or therapy recommendations requires pharmacist counseling under federal law. Technicians may assist with administrative tasks but cannot provide clinical advice. Referral ensures the patient receives accurate, safe medication guidance and maintains compliance with counseling regulations.

Q380. Answer: B

Explanation: RCA focuses on uncovering system-level breakdowns—such as workflow, labeling, or staffing issues—rather than assigning individual blame. This proactive analysis supports process redesign to prevent recurrence. Blame-focused approaches discourage reporting and do not address the true causes of safety events.

Q381. Answer: B

Explanation: The U.S. Food and Drug Administration (FDA) manages MedWatch for voluntary reporting of adverse drug events, product problems, and medication errors. The CDC handles disease surveillance,

ISMP promotes medication-safety education, and the DEA enforces controlled-substance regulations. Reporting through MedWatch enhances pharmacovigilance and product recall awareness.

Q382. Answer: B

Explanation: Technicians must wear appropriate PPE and use a tray exclusively designated for hazardous medications. This prevents residue transfer to non-hazardous drugs. Wiping alone may be inadequate, and pouring drugs back into stock risks contamination and exposure to toxic particles.

Q383. Answer: B

Explanation: Bar-code verification ensures that the correct medication, strength, and patient label are matched, minimizing dispensing errors. While it may indirectly improve communication, its core purpose is automated verification at the dispensing stage. Prescribing and documentation errors originate earlier in the medication-use process.

Q384. Answer: A

Explanation: The abbreviation "U" may resemble a zero or the numeral four, leading to tenfold overdose errors, particularly with insulin or heparin. Writing "unit" in full prevents misinterpretation. Clear, standardized labeling is a cornerstone of safe prescription communication and adherence to ISMP guidelines.

Q385. Answer: B

Explanation: Recalled drugs must be quarantined to prevent dispensing, then managed according to FDA or manufacturer recall instructions. Immediate disposal or continued use violates federal regulations. Proper quarantine ensures traceability and protects patient safety until corrective actions are completed.

Q386. Answer: A

Explanation: An incorrect strength label on the correct product is a labeling error. Wrong drug refers to selection of another medication entirely. Omission involves failure to dispense, and compliance error relates to patient adherence. Labeling errors can cause under- or overdosing if undetected.

Q387. Answer: B

Explanation: Proper hand and forearm washing using antimicrobial soap is the first critical step in aseptic technique. This removes transient microorganisms before gowning and gloving. Cleaning surfaces and gloves follows handwashing, ensuring complete contamination prevention in sterile compounding areas.

Q388. Answer: B

Explanation: CQI programs monitor error rates relative to total prescriptions filled to quantify safety performance. Tracking this ratio identifies trends requiring workflow changes or training. While satisfaction and wait times matter, they are service metrics—not direct patient-safety indicators.

Q389. Answer: B

Explanation: A near-miss should be documented confidentially within the pharmacy's quality-improvement or risk-management system. Reporting helps identify vulnerabilities before harm occurs. External reports like police or insurance are unnecessary unless actual injury or loss is involved. Learning from near misses strengthens prevention strategies.

Q390. Answer: A

Explanation: An allergic response such as hives is an adverse drug event (ADE), even if correctly prescribed. Medication errors involve process mistakes, while noncompliance and storage issues are unrelated. Recording ADEs assists in allergy documentation, pharmacovigilance, and safe future prescribing.

Q391. Answer: B

Explanation: Technicians must refer discrepancies to the pharmacist for professional clarification before contacting the prescriber. Pharmacists evaluate therapeutic intent and communicate appropriately. Independent technician decisions could result in unsafe dispensing or regulatory violations. Always escalate unclear orders to the pharmacist first.

Q392. Answer: B

Explanation: The Occupational Safety and Health Administration (OSHA) enforces workplace safety regulations, including infection-control and hazardous-waste handling standards. The FDA regulates drugs, the DEA controls narcotics, and the CDC provides guidance but not enforcement authority. Compliance ensures staff and patient protection.

Q393. Answer: B

Explanation: Bypassing safety systems undermines error-prevention protocols. Technicians should promptly report such behavior to the pharmacist or supervisor for correction through coaching or retraining. Public confrontation may create conflict, and ignoring it jeopardizes patient safety and regulatory compliance.

Q394. Answer: A

Explanation: Celebrex (celecoxib) and Celexa (citalopram) are LASA drugs that have caused documented confusion. Implementing Tall Man lettering—CeleBREX vs CeLEXA—and separated storage helps prevent mix-ups. Cipro, Ceftin, and Cephalexin are antibiotics with less phonetic similarity, posing lower substitution risk.

Q395. Answer: B

Explanation: Continuous Quality Improvement meetings foster a non-punitive environment for reviewing incidents, identifying patterns, and improving systems. Punitive measures discourage reporting. Staffing limits or quotas do not address root causes and may worsen workload-related risks.

Q396. Answer: B

Explanation: "QD" (once daily) is on the ISMP error-prone abbreviation list because it can be mistaken for "QID." Instead, "daily" should be written in full. BID, PO, and PRN are standard abbreviations accepted in medical communication when written clearly and properly.

Q397. Answer: B

Explanation: Bar-code medication administration (BCMA) ensures correct patient, drug, dose, and time—reducing administration errors. It verifies data before drug administration, minimizing mismatches. Prescribing occurs earlier in the process, while manufacturing and procurement errors are unrelated to bedside administration.

Q398. Answer: C

Explanation: Expired medications must be removed from active inventory and quarantined according to facility and regulatory policies. Relabeling or mixing with new stock violates safety and quality standards. Quarantine prevents accidental dispensing and allows proper return or disposal through authorized channels.

Q399. Answer: B

Explanation: The Institute for Safe Medication Practices (ISMP) develops guidelines to minimize errors, including LASA prevention and Tall Man lettering standards. DEA enforces controlled substances, OSHA handles workplace safety, and CDC focuses on disease prevention rather than medication error strategies.

Q400. Answer: B

Explanation: When an undesired effect occurs despite correct use, it's an adverse drug reaction (ADR). ADRs are not necessarily caused by human error but by drug effects. Dispensing or prescribing errors involve human mistakes, not normal pharmacological reactions like nausea.

Questions (401-500)

Q401. Which hand hygiene practice is required before entering the sterile compounding area?

A. Alcohol rub only

B. Washing hands for 30 seconds with soap and water

C. Rinsing with water only

D. Using lotion before gloves

Q402. A technician notices a coworker preparing an IV admixture without PPE. What should be done immediately?

A. Continue working silently

B. Report to the pharmacist in charge

C. Offer to finish the preparation

D. Document the issue at end of shift

Q403. Which type of error occurs when a technician fails to include the auxiliary label "Shake Well" on a suspension?

A. Compliance error

B. Administration error

C. Wrong drug error

D. Omission error

Q404. The primary goal of Continuous Quality Improvement (CQI) in a pharmacy is to:

A. Punish individual errors

B. Improve workflow and patient safety

C. Reduce technician work hours

D. Eliminate pharmacist counseling

Q405. Which of the following steps should be taken if a technician suspects a dispensing error has occurred?

A. Hide the mistake to avoid discipline

B. Notify the pharmacist immediately

C. Correct it quietly without documentation

D. Discard all evidence

Q406. Which reference source should be used to identify proper infection-control standards in the pharmacy?

A. ISMP

B. USP Chapter <797>

C. DEA Diversion Manual

D. FDA MedWatch

Q407. A technician uses the abbreviation "HS" on a label. What risk does this pose?

A. It can mean "half strength" or "at bedtime"

B. It's an accepted abbreviation

C. It represents "hourly schedule" only

D. It reduces label space

Q408. Which step is required after reporting an adverse drug event to MedWatch?

A. File a police report

B. Notify the prescriber and document internally

C. Send the medication to the manufacturer

D. Destroy the remaining stock immediately

Q409. Which practice helps prevent errors with high-alert medications like heparin?

A. Skipping double-checks to save time

B. Storing separately and labeling clearly
C. Mixing with other drugs for convenience
D. Dispensing from open containers

Q410. What is the best action if a patient brings back medication that appears tampered with?
A. Restock after inspection
B. Accept for return and reuse
C. Quarantine and inform pharmacist
D. Dispose of in regular trash

Q411. Which of the following is the safest labeling instruction for liquid antibiotics?
A. "Store as usual"
B. "Shake well before use and refrigerate"
C. "Do not refrigerate"
D. "Avoid shaking before use"

Q412. A pharmacy technician reports an incident to a Continuous Quality Improvement system. What is this called?
A. Blame report
B. Incident documentation
C. Compliance report
D. Risk assumption form

Q413. Which behavior most supports a culture of safety in the pharmacy?
A. Discouraging reporting to maintain reputation
B. Openly discussing errors to prevent recurrence
C. Penalizing all involved staff
D. Ignoring minor near misses

Q414. Which infection-control step must occur before donning sterile gloves?
A. Clean the hood
B. Wash hands and dry with lint-free towel
C. Spray gloves first with alcohol
D. Inspect gown for tears

Q415. A pharmacy technician mistakenly fills a prescription for metoprolol instead of methyldopa. This is classified as:
A. Wrong drug error
B. Wrong patient error
C. Wrong time error
D. Documentation error

Q416. Which of the following best describes a near miss in pharmacy operations?
A. A medication error that reaches the patient
B. A potential error caught before reaching the patient
C. A misfilled prescription given to the wrong person
D. A documented adverse drug event

Q417. Which auxiliary label is required on all medications that cause drowsiness?
A. "Avoid sunlight."
B. "Take with food."
C. "May cause drowsiness; use caution when operating machinery."
D. "Shake well before use."

Q418. Which of the following is the most effective way to prevent LASA medication errors?
A. Grouping drugs alphabetically
B. Using Tall Man lettering and barcode scanning

C. Placing LASA drugs together for convenience
D. Ignoring differences if packaging is distinct

Q419. During sterile compounding, which surface must be disinfected most frequently?
A. Compounding workbench surface
B. Ceiling vents
C. Storage shelves
D. Pass-through chamber exterior

Q420. A technician records a vaccine error involving incorrect storage temperature. To which system should this be reported?
A. VAERS
B. Medkstch
C. CQI internal log only
D. FDA recall database

Q421. When a technician receives a prescription for a medication outside the pharmacy's usual formulary, what is the safest first step?
A. Substitute a similar medication
B. Dispense the closest alternative
C. Verify with the pharmacist before ordering
D. Refuse and discard the prescription

Q422. What is the main goal of using Tall Man lettering on medication labels?
A. To improve brand recognition
B. To draw attention to differing letter sequences in LASA names
C. To save space on medication labels
D. To simplify printing procedures

Q423. Which of the following describes a sentinel event?
A. A minor documentation error
B. An unexpected event causing serious harm or death
C. A daily process deviation
D. An error corrected before reaching the patient

Q424. Which step ensures sterility in aseptic compounding?
A. Wearing regular gloves
B. Frequent handwashing and use of sterile gloves
C. Using cotton swabs to clean vials
D. Opening all supplies simultaneously

Q425. A technician fills an antibiotic prescription for "500 mg TID × 10 days" but labels it as "BID." Which safety system would best catch this error?
A. Bar-code verification
B. Double-check verification by pharmacist
C. Controlled substance log
D. Manufacturer recall notice

Q426. Which is an example of an administration error?
A. Giving the correct medication to the wrong patient
B. Dispensing expired medication
C. Incorrect transcription of directions
D. Selecting the wrong drug in storage

Q427. What should a technician do immediately after a medication spill in the sterile cleanroom?
A. Continue compounding to avoid delay
B. Stop work and follow facility spill cleanup protocol

C. Mop the spill with paper towels only
D. Ignore small spills under 1 mL

Q428. Which pharmacy workflow feature most reduces medication selection errors?
A. Dim lighting
B. Separate, clearly labeled storage zones
C. Open-shelving layout for all drugs
D. Placing high-alert drugs in front for access

Q429. When documenting a medication error, which information is most important to include?
A. The person at fault
B. The sequence of events and contributing factors
C. Patient insurance information
D. Technician's employment record

Q430. Which of the following practices violates infection prevention protocols?
A. Cleaning counting trays after each use
B. Touching medication with bare hands
C. Using dedicated spatulas for hazardous drugs
D. Wearing gloves when counting antibiotics

Q431. Which agency accredits hospital programs and monitors sentinel events?
A. FDA
B. The Joint Commission
C. CDC
D. ISMP

Q432. A technician is preparing to clean the laminar airflow hood. Which cleaning agent should be used last during the process?
A. Sterile water
B. 70% isopropyl alcohol
C. Bleach solution
D. Soap and water

Q433. What should a technician do if a patient reports dizziness after starting a new antihypertensive medication?
A. Advise stopping immediately
B. Recommend taking with food
C. Refer the patient to the pharmacist
D. Ignore unless symptoms worsen

Q434. Which of the following is the safest way to prevent contamination during nonsterile compounding?
A. Wear gloves and wash hands
B. Use tap water for cleaning
C. Mix directly on open countertop
D. Reuse disposable equipment

Q435. Which label instruction helps prevent photodegradation of light-sensitive medications?
A. Store in freezer
B. Keep container tightly closed
C. Protect from light
D. Shake well before use

Q436. If a technician discovers a temperature deviation in a vaccine refrigerator, what should be done first?
A. Discard all stored vaccines

B. Record the current temperature and notify the pharmacist
C. Reset the thermostat immediately
D. Move vaccines to another fridge without documentation

Q437. Which of the following activities is outside the pharmacy technician's scope?

A. Recording refrigerator temperatures
B. Reporting potential dispensing errors
C. Performing final product verification
D. Cleaning counting trays

Q438. Which type of error occurs when a technician enters the wrong patient profile during prescription processing?

A. Transcription error
B. Dispensing error
C. Administration error
D. Monitoring error

Q439. Which practice minimizes cross-contamination when counting tablets?

A. Using a single spatula for all drugs
B. Cleaning counting trays with alcohol after each use
C. Mixing drugs carefully on same tray
D. Avoiding cleaning unless visible residue appears

Q440. If a technician notices a coworker making repeated data entry mistakes, what is the best course of action?

A. Ignore it to avoid conflict
B. Report patterns to the supervising pharmacist
C. Correct entries silently without documentation
D. Discuss errors with other technicians

Q441. A patient's prescription is labeled "Take one tablet QID," but the prescriber intended "QD." What kind of error is this?

A. Transcription
B. Abbreviation misinterpretation
C. Dispensing
D. Omission

Q442. What should be done immediately if a technician spills a hazardous drug solution?

A. Leave it until end of shift
B. Wipe with paper towels only
C. Use a spill kit and notify supervisor
D. Rinse with tap water

Q443. Which scenario demonstrates an omission error?

A. Wrong drug chosen from shelf
B. Missing dose not given to patient
C. Label printed with incorrect strength
D. Duplicate medication filled

Q444. What is the primary purpose of error reporting systems like MedWatch and CQI logs?

A. To punish responsible staff
B. To identify trends and prevent recurrence
C. To reduce staffing levels
D. To report only fatal events

Q445. Which practice prevents wrong-patient medication errors?

A. Using at least two unique patient identifiers

B. Asking only for the patient's first name
C. Skipping verification during refills
D. Matching medication color only

Q446. When compounding hazardous drugs, which engineering control provides the greatest protection to personnel?
A. Laminar airflow workbench
B. Biological safety cabinet (Class II)
C. Regular countertop workspace
D. Refrigerator with exhaust vent

Q447. A technician receives a prescription written as ".5 mg" instead of "0.5 mg." Why is this format unsafe?
A. It can be mistaken as 5 mg
B. It wastes label space
C. It is stylistically incorrect
D. It's not required under DEA law

Q448. Which measure best prevents calculation-related medication errors?
A. Mental math when busy
B. Double-checking calculations with a second verifier
C. Estimating doses using experience
D. Ignoring small discrepancies

Q449. Which process ensures that expired medications are removed and not dispensed?
A. FIFO rotation system
B. Random stock checks
C. Quarterly audits only
D. Verbal reminders

Q450. What is the correct procedure if a prescription error results in patient harm?
A. Delete the record immediately
B. Notify the pharmacist and complete incident documentation
C. Attempt to fix the record quietly
D. Wait until the patient files a complaint

Q451. A patient receives a duplicate refill for a discontinued drug. This should be classified as which type of error?
A. Wrong dose error
B. Compliance error
C. Wrong drug error
D. Monitoring error

Q452. A technician notices that a controlled medication count is short. What should be done first?
A. Adjust the count in the computer
B. Notify the pharmacist immediately
C. Reorder stock silently
D. Ignore unless discrepancy persists

Q453. Which safety step must be taken before transferring a patient's prescription to another pharmacy?
A. Discard the original prescription
B. Verify transfer eligibility and record details accurately
C. Call the insurance company
D. Fill both copies to ensure coverage

Q454. Which infection control measure reduces contamination during aseptic compounding?

A. Wearing jewelry under gloves
B. Disinfecting vials before needle entry
C. Talking over the hood during work
D. Using torn gowns

Q455. Which of the following actions would most likely reduce prescription labeling errors?
A. Allowing multitasking during verification
B. Skipping patient confirmation
C. Rushing during peak hours
D. Using barcode label verification systems

Q456. Which of the following represents an unsafe abbreviation?
A. mcg
B. IU
C. mEq
D. mL

Q457. When preparing chemotherapy agents, which personal protective equipment (PPE) must always be worn?
A. Gloves only
B. Gown, gloves, and face shield
C. Regular mask only
D. Apron only

Q458. Which of the following incidents must be reported to MedWatch?
A. Incorrect dose dispensed but corrected before use
B. Adverse reaction to an FDA-approved medication
C. Minor packaging color change
D. Routine vaccine administration

Q459. A prescription label for warfarin lacks the "Caution: High Alert Medication" auxiliary label. This error is categorized as:
A. Wrong drug
B. Documentation error
C. Administration error
D. Labeling error

Q460. Why should medications not be poured back into stock bottles once dispensed?
A. It wastes product
B. It may cause contamination
C. It's time-consuming
D. It voids insurance claims

Q461. A technician discovers a potential drug interaction in the patient profile. What is the appropriate next step?
A. Ignore and continue filling
B. Alert the pharmacist immediately
C. Ask the patient for medical advice
D. Dispense with a warning label

Q462. What is the correct procedure if a technician experiences a needle stick while compounding?
A. Rinse and continue working
B. Report immediately and follow exposure protocol
C. Hide incident to avoid documentation
D. Dispose of gloves and ignore

Q463. Which example illustrates a "look-alike/sound-alike" (LASA) drug pair?

A. Metformin and Methadone
B. Amoxicillin and Ampicillin
C. Hydralazine and Hydroxyzine
D. Atenolol and Atorvastatin

Q464. Which factor most increases the likelihood of a medication error?
A. Clear labeling
B. Distractions and interruptions
C. Using barcode systems
D. Double verification

Q465. Which type of error involves dispensing medication to the wrong patient?
A. Wrong patient error
B. Wrong dose error
C. Wrong time error
D. Documentation error

Q466. How often should HEPA filters in a cleanroom be certified according to USP <797>?
A. Monthly
B. Every 6 months
C. Annually
D. Every 2 years

Q467. Which step ensures traceability in compounding documentation?
A. Recording lot numbers and expiration dates of all ingredients
B. Discarding worksheets after completion
C. Using generic product descriptions
D. Skipping signature fields

Q468. Which of the following is a pharmacist-only responsibility?
A. Conducting final product verification
B. Counting tablets
C. Cleaning compounding area
D. Entering prescription data

Q469. What should be done if a controlled substance prescription appears altered?
A. Fill only part of it
B. Notify the pharmacist for verification
C. Call the patient for clarification
D. Ignore and process normally

Q470. A technician observes a pharmacist entering the sterile cleanroom without performing hand hygiene. What is the proper response?
A. Ignore it, assuming expertise
B. Immediately remind and report through safety channels
C. Document anonymously only
D. Wait until the end of the shift

Q471. Which of the following actions violates USP <797> aseptic compounding standards?
A. Cleaning hood with 70% isopropyl alcohol
B. Wearing artificial nails while compounding
C. Using sterile gloves
D. Cleaning workbench between batches

Q472. What type of error occurs when a patient's allergy information is not entered into the computer system?
A. Omission error

B. Wrong drug error
C. Documentation error
D. Compliance error

Q473. A patient experiences excessive bleeding after taking warfarin and aspirin together. This event is best described as:

A. Drug interaction
B. Dispensing error
C. Labeling error
D. Compliance error

Q474. A technician notices multiple LASA drugs stored alphabetically next to each other. What is the best action?

A. Leave them as they are
B. Separate and label using Tall Man lettering
C. Color-code bottles by manufacturer
D. Store all LASA drugs on the same shelf

Q475. What should a technician do if a patient questions why their medication looks different than before?

A. Say it's the same and move on
B. Refer the patient to the pharmacist
C. Tell them generics often look identical
D. Replace it without checking

Q476. Which statement about high-alert medications is true?

A. They have no special handling requirements
B. They require extra verification before dispensing
C. They are only used in hospitals
D. They are not listed by ISMP

Q477. Which of the following scenarios qualifies as a "sentinel event"?

A. Wrong label printed but corrected
B. Delayed refill
C. Death caused by medication mix-up
D. Missing auxiliary label

Q478. When preparing an IV admixture, where should the technician position hands inside the laminar airflow hood?

A. In front of the HEPA filter
B. Away from critical airflow zone
C. Upstream of sterile airflow
D. Directly in airflow path between HEPA filter and product

Q479. What is the technician's responsibility during pharmacist verification?

A. Provide complete, accurate preparation and documentation
B. Sign off on the prescription
C. Counsel the patient about therapy
D. Change directions if unclear

Q480. Which behavior demonstrates a culture of safety in pharmacy practice?

A. Concealing near misses
B. Encouraging open reporting without punishment
C. Discouraging communication with management
D. Ignoring system flaws

Q481. Which infection prevention procedure is required between glove changes in sterile compounding?
A. Wash hands again completely
B. Spray new gloves with 70% isopropyl alcohol
C. Skip disinfection for time efficiency
D. Touch surrounding surfaces for balance
Q482. Which practice best prevents cross-contamination between hazardous and nonhazardous medications?
A. Shared counting trays
B. Separate equipment and work areas
C. Wiping all drugs with alcohol
D. Rotating tools daily
Q483. What is the recommended cleaning order for surfaces in a laminar hood?
A. Front to back, top to bottom
B. Back to front, top to bottom
C. Random pattern for coverage
D. Circular wiping motion
Q484. Which of the following must be included in every medication error report?
A. Names of all pharmacy staff
B. Store sales for the day
C. Patient's insurance provider
D. Description of event and contributing factors
Q485. A technician notices a coworker falsifying refrigerator temperature logs. What is the most appropriate action?
A. Correct it silently
B. Report the falsification to the pharmacist or supervisor
C. Ignore to avoid confrontation
D. Change the record back later
Q486. Which organization publishes the "Do Not Use" abbreviation list?
A. DEA
B. The Joint Commission
C. FDA
D. OSHA
Q487. When a patient reports a mild rash after taking an antibiotic, the technician should:
A. Recommend an antihistamine
B. Refer immediately to the pharmacist
C. Ignore unless severe
D. Advise discontinuing and throwing away all medication
Q488. Which safety measure helps reduce transcription errors during prescription entry?
A. Using drop-down lists and bar-code scanning
B. Relying on memory for common drugs
C. Entering prescriptions quickly to save time
D. Ignoring alert prompts
Q489. Which of the following is a key element of a Continuous Quality Improvement (CQI) plan?
A. Root-cause analysis and preventive actions
B. Assigning individual blame
C. Minimizing documentation
D. Skipping minor errors

Q490. Which practice minimizes medication errors when entering verbal prescriptions?
A. Enter quickly to save time
B. Repeat the order back to the prescriber
C. Ask another technician to confirm
D. Skip patient verification
Q491. A patient's antibiotic was labeled "Take 1 tablet every 4 hours," but the order said "every 6 hours." What type of error is this?
A. Wrong patient error
B. Wrong dose error
C. Wrong frequency error
D. Omission error
Q492. Which step should always be performed before opening ampules during compounding?
A. Wipe with 70% isopropyl alcohol
B. Tap to break without cleaning
C. Wipe with water
D. Shake vigorously
Q493. Which documentation should be completed when a technician accidentally prepares the wrong IV solution?
A. Discard silently
B. Record in the CQI incident log
C. Notify prescriber only
D. Reuse solution for another patient
Q494. What is the safest action when a patient insists on taking an expired prescription medication?
A. Advise disposal and refer to pharmacist
B. Allow use if recently expired
C. Reprint label with a new date
D. Provide reassurance it's still potent
Q495. Which control measure helps ensure accuracy in sterile compounding calculations?
A. Rounding to the nearest gram
B. Independent verification by another technician
C. Estimating doses visually
D. Using handwritten math notes only
Q496. What should a technician do if a vial of insulin is found stored at room temperature beyond its allowable period?
A. Reuse until color changes
B. Return to the refrigerator
C. Quarantine and inform the pharmacist
D. Dispense to avoid waste
Q497. Which of the following is an example of an environmental control in quality assurance?
A. Staff training
B. Airflow certification of cleanroom
C. Label verification
D. Error reporting meeting
Q498. A technician fills an order for "morphine 15 mg" but selects "hydromorphone 2 mg" instead. This represents:
A. Wrong strength error
B. Wrong drug error
C. Transcription error

D. Compliance error

Q499. Which of the following abbreviations is prohibited because it can be mistaken for "0"?

A. U

B. mcg

C. mL

D. mg

Q500. A technician finds particulate matter in a reconstituted suspension. What should be done?

A. Dispense if label matches

B. Shake vigorously and dispense

C. Discard and prepare a new suspension

D. Filter and relabel

Answer key and Explanation (401-500)

Q401. Answer: B

Explanation: Handwashing with antimicrobial soap and warm water for at least 30 seconds removes microorganisms and prevents contamination during aseptic compounding. Alcohol rubs are supplemental, not replacements. Lotions can compromise glove integrity, and rinsing alone does not meet sterile standards.

Q402. Answer: B

Explanation: PPE noncompliance in sterile compounding presents contamination risk. The technician must promptly inform the supervising pharmacist to halt unsafe practice and retrain staff. Continuing work or delaying reporting enables further safety breaches and violates USP <797> standards.

Q403. Answer: D

Explanation: Missing a required label is an omission error—a failure to perform a necessary task. This can lead to improper use of suspensions, reducing efficacy. Wrong drug and administration errors involve different steps, and compliance errors pertain to patient adherence.

Q404. Answer: B

Explanation: CQI focuses on system improvement to prevent errors and enhance safety. It encourages team learning, documentation, and process evaluation. Punishment undermines error reporting. CQI does not reduce staffing or eliminate counseling, both of which are essential to quality assurance.

Q405. Answer: B

Explanation: The technician must report suspected errors to the pharmacist for immediate assessment and patient protection. Concealing or altering evidence breaches ethical and legal standards. Prompt reporting allows corrective action, error analysis, and transparency under CQI principles.

Q406. Answer: B

Explanation: USP Chapter <797> outlines sterile compounding standards, including aseptic technique, garbing, and environmental control. ISMP handles error prevention, DEA addresses controlled substances, and MedWatch reports adverse drug events—not infection control specifics. Adherence ensures sterile product safety.

Q407. Answer: A

Explanation: "HS" is dangerous because it can mean "half strength" or "at bedtime," leading to misinterpretation. The term should be written out fully to prevent dosing confusion. Clarity in labeling and directions supports patient understanding and minimizes medication errors.

Q408. Answer: B

Explanation: After submitting a MedWatch report, internal documentation and prescriber notification ensure continuity of care and record accuracy. Destroying or returning drugs is not required unless directed by recall. Coordination between pharmacy and prescriber strengthens pharmacovigilance practices.

Q409. Answer: B

Explanation: High-alert drugs should be isolated in storage with clear labels and double-verification procedures to prevent dosing errors. Combining or using unsealed containers increases contamination and selection risk. Organized separation aligns with ISMP and USP safety recommendations.

Q410. Answer: C

Explanation: Returned or tampered medications must be quarantined until evaluated by the pharmacist for possible DEA-compliant disposal. Reuse or restocking violates safety laws and increases contamination risk. Regular trash disposal endangers the public and breaches hazardous waste regulations.

Q411. Answer: B

Explanation: Most reconstituted antibiotics require refrigeration and thorough shaking to maintain stability and uniform dose distribution. Incorrect storage or neglecting agitation may reduce potency. "Shake well before use and refrigerate" ensures consistent dosing and effective antimicrobial action.

Q412. Answer: B

Explanation: Incident documentation is a formal CQI record used to analyze, not punish, errors or near misses. It helps improve procedures and prevent recurrence. Compliance and risk forms address regulations or liability, not internal safety reporting.

Q413. Answer: B

Explanation: Open, blame-free discussion promotes continuous improvement and transparency. Staff learn collectively and reinforce preventive measures. Suppressing reports or punishing staff fosters fear, while ignoring near misses misses vital learning opportunities. A strong safety culture encourages accountability and collaboration.

Q414. Answer: B

Explanation: Proper handwashing and drying prevent microbial transfer to gloves. Performing this before gloving is essential to maintain asepsis in sterile compounding. Cleaning the hood and inspecting gowns are separate preparation steps. Alcohol spraying follows gloving, not before.

Q415. Answer: A

Explanation: Substituting one drug for another constitutes a wrong drug error. Both names sound similar but have distinct indications. Accurate drug selection, barcode use, and LASA precautions prevent such errors. Documentation or timing issues occur in different process stages.

Q416. Answer: B

Explanation: A near miss is an error intercepted before reaching the patient, offering an opportunity for system improvement. Recording and analyzing near misses enhances quality and reduces future incidents. If the medication reaches the patient, it becomes a reportable medication error or adverse event.

Q417. Answer: C

Explanation: Drowsy-causing medications like antihistamines or opioids require cautionary labels to alert patients about impaired alertness. "Take with food" or "shake well" apply to other categories, while "avoid sunlight" is for photosensitizing agents. Proper labeling promotes safe self-administration and compliance.

Q418. Answer: B

Explanation: Combining Tall Man lettering (e.g., hydrOXYzine vs hydrALAZINE) with barcode verification is a proven safety strategy to prevent LASA errors. Alphabetical grouping or visual recognition alone is insufficient. ISMP recommends both labeling and technology safeguards for best results.

Q419. Answer: A

Explanation: The compounding workbench, or primary engineering control, must be cleaned and disinfected frequently—before and after each use—to maintain aseptic conditions. Surfaces like vents and shelves require scheduled cleaning, but the work area poses the highest contamination risk.

Q420. Answer: A

Explanation: Vaccine-related errors and adverse reactions are reported to the Vaccine Adverse Event Reporting System (VAERS). MedWatch applies to non-vaccine drug events. Internal CQI logs support documentation, but VAERS provides centralized national surveillance for immunization-related incidents.

Q421. Answer: C

Explanation: The technician must alert the pharmacist to evaluate therapeutic alternatives or ordering options before dispensing. Unauthorized substitutions can result in errors or legal issues. Pharmacist verification ensures accurate therapy selection and adherence to state and federal law.

Q422. Answer: B

Explanation: Tall Man lettering highlights distinct portions of LASA drug names (e.g., predniSONE vs prednisoLONE), reducing confusion during selection. It enhances visual differentiation without changing meaning. It is a safety measure promoted by ISMP, not a marketing tool.

Q423. Answer: B

Explanation: Sentinel events result in serious injury or death and trigger immediate root-cause analysis. They reveal critical system failures needing urgent correction. Minor or intercepted errors do not qualify. The Joint Commission mandates investigation and corrective action after such events.

Q424. Answer: B

Explanation: Aseptic integrity depends on hand hygiene and use of sterile gloves to prevent contamination. Regular gloves lack sterility. Cotton swabs and uncoordinated workflow introduce contaminants. Following USP <797> standards guarantees a sterile environment during compounding.

Q425. Answer: B

Explanation: Pharmacist verification provides the final checkpoint to detect dosage or labeling discrepancies before dispensing. Bar-code systems verify drug identity, not directions. Controlled logs and recall notices are unrelated. Multiple human and technological checks enhance patient safety.

Q426. Answer: A

Explanation: Administration errors occur during delivery to the patient—such as giving the correct drug to the wrong person or at the wrong time. Dispensing, transcription, and selection errors occur earlier in the medication-use process, typically within pharmacy workflow.

Q427. Answer: B

Explanation: All spills, regardless of volume, require immediate cleanup per hazardous or non-hazardous protocols to prevent contamination and exposure. Continuing work violates USP standards. Only trained personnel should handle cleanups using PPE and proper disinfectants.

Q428. Answer: B

Explanation: Distinct, well-labeled storage areas reduce confusion, especially for LASA and high-alert medications. Adequate lighting and proper shelf organization are core safety standards. Open or high-traffic access areas increase misselection risk and compromise inventory control.

Q429. Answer: B

Explanation: Effective documentation should focus on objective details—what occurred, when, and contributing system factors. Blame or personal details do not improve prevention. Understanding workflow context supports RCA and CQI initiatives to enhance pharmacy safety practices.

Q430. Answer: B

Explanation: Handling medications with bare hands risks contamination and exposure. Gloves and dedicated tools maintain hygiene and protect both technician and patient. Regular cleaning of trays further prevents cross-contamination between different medications.

Q431. Answer: B

Explanation: The Joint Commission accredits healthcare organizations and requires reporting and investigation of sentinel events. It promotes continuous improvement in patient safety and quality care. FDA regulates drugs, CDC monitors disease, and ISMP provides error-prevention resources, not accreditation.

Q432. Answer: B

Explanation: Final disinfection of the laminar hood must use 70% isopropyl alcohol, applied after removal of residue with sterile water. Alcohol provides rapid microbial kill and evaporates cleanly. Bleach and soap may corrode surfaces and are not part of final aseptic cleaning.

Q433. Answer: C

Explanation: Technicians must refer any report of side effects, such as dizziness, to the pharmacist for clinical assessment. They may not provide medical advice or modify therapy. Early referral ensures safe evaluation for dose adjustment or counseling.

Q434. Answer: A

Explanation: Wearing gloves and practicing hand hygiene prevent introduction of contaminants during nonsterile compounding. Tap water may contain impurities, and open countertops or reused equipment introduce microbial or particulate contamination, compromising product quality and patient safety.

Q435. Answer: C

Explanation: "Protect from light" prevents photochemical degradation that reduces potency in drugs like nitroprusside or amphotericin. Light exposure can alter chemical structure. Other instructions serve different purposes such as maintaining sterility or suspension uniformity, not photoprotection.

Q436. Answer: B

Explanation: Documenting the deviation and informing the pharmacist ensures appropriate assessment before use or disposal. Immediate thermostat changes may conceal evidence. Vaccine integrity must be evaluated based on stability data and manufacturer guidance, ensuring safety and compliance.

Q437. Answer: C

Explanation: Final verification is restricted to licensed pharmacists. Technicians assist with quality control but cannot legally perform final checks. Temperature logs, reporting errors, and cleaning duties are technician responsibilities that support safe pharmacy operations.

Q438. Answer: A

Explanation: Selecting or entering data into the wrong patient profile is a transcription error, arising from inaccurate data entry. Dispensing errors occur later during product selection or labeling. Administration and monitoring errors happen after dispensing or during therapy.

Q439. Answer: B

Explanation: Counting trays and spatulas must be cleaned with alcohol after every use to prevent residue transfer between medications. Cross-contamination can cause allergic reactions or therapeutic errors. Using one tool for all products violates hygiene protocols.

Q440. Answer: B

Explanation: Reporting repeated mistakes to the supervising pharmacist allows corrective action, such as retraining or workflow review. Ignoring or gossiping fails to resolve safety risks. Proper communication channels preserve confidentiality and protect patient outcomes.

Q441. Answer: B

Explanation: Confusion between "QD" (daily) and "QID" (four times daily) is a classic abbreviation misinterpretation error. Such mistakes underscore the need to write "daily" or "four times daily" to avoid ambiguity. Eliminating unsafe abbreviations is central to error prevention.

Q442. Answer: C

Explanation: Hazardous drug spills require containment with a designated spill kit and supervisor notification. PPE and proper disposal prevent exposure and contamination. Improvised cleanup without containment violates USP <800> safety requirements and endangers staff health.

Q443. Answer: B

Explanation: An omission error occurs when a required medication dose is missed or not administered. It differs from selection or labeling errors. Omission may lead to therapeutic failure or adverse effects, emphasizing adherence monitoring and communication.

Q444. Answer: B

Explanation: Reporting systems identify trends, root causes, and patterns to improve systems and prevent future incidents. They are designed for safety learning, not punishment. Limiting reports to severe events undermines continuous improvement and reduces detection of systemic weaknesses.

Q445. Answer: A

Explanation: Verifying two identifiers, such as name and date of birth, ensures correct patient matching before dispensing. Relying on single identifiers or appearance risks mix-ups, especially in busy or multi-patient environments. Consistent verification reduces patient harm.

Q446. Answer: B

Explanation: A Class II Biological Safety Cabinet protects both the compounder and the environment from exposure. Laminar hoods protect only the product. Regular counters lack containment, and refrigerators aren't designed for manipulation of hazardous drugs.

Q447. Answer: A

Explanation: A missing leading zero may result in a tenfold overdose if ".5 mg" is misread as "5 mg." The use of leading zeros before decimal points ensures clarity and aligns with ISMP safe medication practices.

Q448. Answer: B

Explanation: Independent double-checks for all calculations, especially for pediatric and high-alert drugs, significantly reduce risk. Mental math and estimation invite errors. Verifying independently ensures both accuracy and accountability in dose preparation.

Q449. Answer: A

Explanation: The First-In, First-Out (FIFO) system ensures older stock is used first, preventing expiration before dispensing. It's part of pharmacy inventory control and regulatory compliance. Random checks and reminders are less reliable for maintaining product integrity.

Q450. Answer: B

Explanation: Immediate notification of the pharmacist and detailed documentation ensures legal and ethical compliance. Transparency allows investigation, error correction, and patient follow-up. Concealing or delaying reports can worsen outcomes and violate state board and institutional reporting requirements.

Q451. Answer: D

Explanation: Dispensing a discontinued medication reflects a monitoring error, as therapy status was not properly reviewed. Monitoring ensures current therapy appropriateness. Wrong drug and dose refer to incorrect selections, while compliance errors involve patient behavior post-dispensing.

Q452. Answer: B

Explanation: Controlled substance discrepancies must be reported to the pharmacist for prompt investigation and reconciliation. Adjusting counts independently can be considered tampering. Reporting ensures compliance with DEA requirements and helps detect diversion or counting errors early.

Q453. Answer: B

Explanation: Before transferring, technicians must verify eligibility (refill status, controlled classification) and document details—dates, pharmacist names, and prescription numbers—to comply with federal law. Double filling or discarding originals violates transfer and recordkeeping regulations.

Q454. Answer: B

Explanation: Disinfecting vial stoppers with 70% isopropyl alcohol before puncture removes microorganisms that could enter sterile preparations. Jewelry, speaking, or improper PPE compromise asepsis and increase contamination risk. Strict aseptic discipline ensures sterility and patient safety.

Q455. Answer: D

Explanation: Barcode verification ensures that printed labels correspond to the correct drug, dose, and patient. It automates verification, minimizing transcription or printing errors. Multitasking, rushing, or omitting patient checks increases labeling inaccuracy.

Q456. Answer: B

Explanation: "IU" (International Units) can be mistaken for "IV" or "10," leading to overdoses. It should be written as "units." The other abbreviations—mcg, mEq, and mL—are considered standard and safe according to ISMP recommendations.

Q457. Answer: B

Explanation: Handling hazardous drugs such as chemotherapy agents requires a protective gown, double gloves, and face or eye protection to prevent dermal and mucosal exposure. Single PPE pieces do not provide adequate protection per USP <800> standards.

Q458. Answer: B

Explanation: MedWatch collects reports of adverse reactions, medication errors, and quality problems involving FDA-regulated products. Non-adverse events like minor labeling or packaging changes are not reportable unless they affect safety or efficacy.

Q459. Answer: D

Explanation: Missing required cautionary labeling is a labeling error, potentially leading to improper handling or dosing. High-alert drugs like warfarin require clear warnings due to their narrow therapeutic index. Correct labeling prevents serious adverse events.

Q460. Answer: B

Explanation: Once medication leaves the pharmacy's control, sterility and integrity cannot be guaranteed. Returning dispensed medication risks contamination and violates state and federal regulations. Instead, such products should be quarantined or destroyed per policy.

Q461. Answer: B

Explanation: Identifying potential drug interactions requires immediate pharmacist review for clinical decision-making. Technicians cannot assess therapeutic relevance. Early intervention prevents harm and upholds the pharmacist's verification responsibilities for drug interaction checks.

Q462. Answer: B

Explanation: Any occupational exposure or needle stick must be reported immediately for medical evaluation and documentation per OSHA and facility safety policies. Prompt reporting ensures timely prophylaxis and compliance with worker-safety standards.

Q463. Answer: C

Explanation: Hydralazine (antihypertensive) and Hydroxyzine (antihistamine) have similar names and packaging, making them LASA drugs. These require Tall Man lettering and separation to avoid selection errors. Others may share prefixes but are not high-risk LASA pairs.

Q464. Answer: B

Explanation: Frequent interruptions and multitasking increase cognitive load and reduce focus, making errors more likely. Minimizing distractions through structured workflow improves safety and accuracy in dispensing.

Q465. Answer: A

Explanation: Delivering medication to the incorrect individual is a wrong patient error, often caused by poor verification. Using two identifiers (name and date of birth) prevents such incidents. Other options involve timing or record inaccuracies.

Q466. Answer: B

Explanation: USP <797> requires HEPA filters to be tested and certified at least every six months or after relocation or maintenance. Regular verification ensures airflow integrity and contamination control in sterile environments.

Q467. Answer: A

Explanation: Traceability relies on detailed recording of lot numbers, quantities, and expiration dates. This allows recall tracking and verification of ingredient sources. Skipping or discarding records breaks compliance and audit trails.

Q468. Answer: A

Explanation: Only licensed pharmacists may perform final verification to ensure therapeutic accuracy and legal compliance. Technicians handle preparation, data entry, and maintenance tasks under supervision. Final check authority cannot be delegated.

Q469. Answer: B

Explanation: Any suspected alteration or forgery must be referred immediately to the pharmacist, who will verify with the prescriber or law enforcement if needed. Technicians cannot modify or process suspicious prescriptions.

Q470. Answer: B

Explanation: All personnel, regardless of title, must follow aseptic protocol. Hand hygiene violations can cause contamination. Prompt, respectful reminder and documentation through safety channels maintain sterile integrity and reinforce accountability under USP <797>.

Q471. Answer: B

Explanation: Artificial nails harbor microorganisms and cannot be adequately disinfected, making them prohibited in sterile compounding environments. Gloves and alcohol cleaning promote sterility. Noncompliance with grooming standards increases the risk of microbial contamination.

Q472. Answer: C

Explanation: Failing to record critical information like allergies represents a documentation error, which can later lead to adverse events. Omission errors relate to missing medication doses, while compliance errors reflect patient adherence. Proper documentation supports safety and clinical decision-making.

Q473. Answer: A

Explanation: The combination of warfarin and aspirin increases bleeding risk due to additive anticoagulant effects—a drug interaction. Dispensing and labeling may have been correct, but this clinical reaction underscores the importance of interaction checks during profile review.

Q474. Answer: B

Explanation: Separating LASA drugs and using Tall Man lettering minimizes mix-ups. Alphabetical or manufacturer grouping increases confusion risk. Visual differentiation is essential for error prevention and aligns with ISMP recommendations.

Q475. Answer: B

Explanation: Any patient concern about medication appearance requires pharmacist review to confirm legitimacy and counsel. Changes may stem from generic substitutions but can also indicate dispensing errors. Referral ensures verification and patient reassurance.

Q476. Answer: B

Explanation: High-alert medications, such as insulin, anticoagulants, and opioids, demand independent double-checks due to their narrow safety margin. ISMP maintains the official list. Extra handling steps prevent catastrophic patient harm from dosing errors.

Q477. Answer: C

Explanation: A sentinel event involves unexpected patient death or severe injury from a healthcare process failure, such as a drug mix-up. It requires immediate root-cause analysis and corrective action. Minor errors corrected early are not sentinel events.

Q478. Answer: D

Explanation: Hands must remain within the direct airflow path between the HEPA filter and product to preserve sterile conditions. Blocking airflow with hands or objects disrupts laminar flow and introduces contaminants. Proper positioning maintains asepsis.

Q479. Answer: A

Explanation: The technician ensures all labeling, preparation, and data entry are correct and ready for pharmacist verification. Pharmacists conduct final checks and counseling. Technicians must not alter directions but provide full, accurate work for review.

Q480. Answer: B

Explanation: A safety culture promotes open reporting and continuous learning without blame. Staff freely identify hazards, supporting CQI processes. Concealment and punitive approaches suppress transparency and hinder prevention of future errors.

Q481. Answer: B

Explanation: Before resuming work, technicians must sanitize new sterile gloves with 70% isopropyl alcohol to maintain asepsis. Handwashing is reserved for before gowning, not between glove changes. Touching non-sterile surfaces compromises sterility.

Q482. Answer: B

Explanation: Dedicated equipment and segregated work areas prevent residue transfer from hazardous to nonhazardous medications. Shared or rotating tools risk contamination and violate USP <800> containment standards. Alcohol wiping alone is insufficient.

Q483. Answer: B

Explanation: Cleaning should proceed back to front and top to bottom to move contaminants away from the HEPA filter and prevent recontamination. Consistent directionality ensures full surface coverage and aseptic compliance per USP <797>.

Q484. Answer: D

Explanation: Effective reports document event details, contributing causes, and corrective measures. Identifying personal blame or unrelated data adds no safety value. Comprehensive documentation supports RCA and CQI programs for error reduction.

Q485. Answer: B

Explanation: Falsifying safety records endangers compliance and product integrity. Reporting through proper channels allows corrective action and maintains legal accountability. Silent corrections or ignoring misconduct perpetuate risk and ethical violations.

Q486. Answer: B

Explanation: The Joint Commission mandates the "Do Not Use" abbreviation list to prevent misinterpretation of medication orders. It standardizes safe communication across healthcare settings. The FDA, DEA, and OSHA focus on regulation, not documentation standards.

Q487. Answer: B

Explanation: Any allergic reaction, regardless of severity, must be reported to the pharmacist for assessment and potential prescriber notification. Technicians may not provide clinical advice or treatment recommendations. Early referral prevents escalation and ensures appropriate management.

Q488. Answer: A

Explanation: Electronic entry systems with drop-down lists and bar-code scanning minimize manual typing and name confusion. Speeding through entry or dismissing alerts increases error likelihood. Automation supports accuracy and workflow safety.

Q489. Answer: A

Explanation: CQI emphasizes root-cause analysis, corrective actions, and ongoing monitoring to prevent recurrence. It treats errors as learning opportunities rather than blame events. Dismissing minor incidents undermines the system's goal of comprehensive safety improvement.

Q490. Answer: B

Explanation: Repeating verbal orders ensures accuracy by confirming the medication name, strength, dose, and directions. It reduces misunderstanding caused by similar-sounding words. This "read-back" technique is endorsed by ISMP and Joint Commission as a best safety practice.

Q491. Answer: C

Explanation: Incorrect frequency—dispensing with directions every 4 hours instead of 6—is a wrong frequency error. It alters the therapeutic interval, increasing toxicity or decreasing efficacy. Wrong dose refers to strength mislabeling, and omission involves missing doses.

Q492. Answer: A

Explanation: Ampules must be wiped with 70% isopropyl alcohol to remove contaminants before snapping open. This prevents glass or particulate contamination in sterile preparations. Water is ineffective, and shaking may cause breakage or injury.

Q493. Answer: B

Explanation: All compounding errors must be logged in the Continuous Quality Improvement (CQI) or event reporting system. This record supports analysis and prevention of recurrence. Discarding without documentation hides valuable safety data and breaches compliance.

Q494. Answer: A

Explanation: Expired drugs may lose potency or become unsafe. Technicians must instruct proper disposal and refer the patient to the pharmacist for counseling. Reprinting or authorizing use violates pharmacy law and endangers the patient.

Q495. Answer: B

Explanation: Independent double-checks by another qualified person verify both math and preparation steps. Visual or handwritten estimation invites significant errors, especially for high-risk drugs. Two-person verification is a USP <797> best practice.

Q496. Answer: C

Explanation: Insulin stability decreases after prolonged room-temperature exposure. It must be quarantined and evaluated by the pharmacist. Returning to refrigeration does not restore potency, and dispensing compromised insulin violates safety standards.

Q497. Answer: B

Explanation: Environmental controls include maintaining and certifying laminar airflow systems to ensure proper air quality for sterile compounding. Staff training and error reviews are administrative, not environmental, measures. Clean airflow prevents contamination and supports aseptic safety.

Q498. Answer: B

Explanation: Substituting a completely different medication, even with similar packaging, is a wrong drug error. Morphine and hydromorphone differ significantly in potency. Proper barcode verification and visual double-checks help prevent this dangerous mistake.

Q499. Answer: A

Explanation: The abbreviation "U" for "unit" can be misread as "0" or "4," causing tenfold dosing errors. Writing "unit" in full ensures clarity. The others—mcg, mL, and mg—are standard metric notations.

Q500. Answer: C

Explanation: The presence of particulate matter indicates contamination or instability; the product must be discarded and remade. Filtering or shaking doesn't ensure sterility or quality. Preparing a fresh suspension guarantees patient safety and product integrity.

Questions (501-600)

Q501. Which of the following demonstrates an error-prevention strategy?
A. Skipping verification for routine drugs
B. Using standardized order forms and labeling
C. Ignoring minor discrepancies
D. Relying solely on technician memory

Q502. What is the technician's role after a medication error has been verified?
A. Identify fault and assign blame
B. Complete documentation and assist in RCA
C. Discuss details with the patient directly
D. Modify the patient's therapy

Q503. Which practice improves patient understanding and reduces administration errors?
A. Providing written and verbal counseling by the pharmacist
B. Giving abbreviated labels only
C. Using technical jargon
D. Limiting instructions to dosage form

Q504. Which of the following requires wearing a respirator mask during cleanup?
A. Liquid antibiotic spill
B. Cytotoxic chemotherapy spill
C. Reconstituted oral suspension spill
D. Normal saline spill

Q505. What is the recommended action if an unlabeled IV admixture bag is found in the refrigerator?
A. Discard immediately per policy
B. Label based on memory
C. Verify and relabel if possible
D. Assume it's saline

Q506. Which medication would typically carry a "High Alert" auxiliary label?
A. Amoxicillin
B. Warfarin
C. Loratadine
D. Acetaminophen

Q507. A technician accidentally skips the final verification step before dispensing. What kind of error risk does this create?
A. Process omission error
B. Wrong patient error
C. Wrong strength error
D. Documentation error

Q508. Which safety measure helps prevent contamination during sterile compounding?
A. Wearing sterile gloves over unwashed hands
B. Avoiding jewelry and cosmetics
C. Keeping supplies open between batches
D. Touching critical surfaces when adjusting items

Q509. When documenting an adverse event, what should be avoided?
A. Objective facts
B. Emotional or subjective statements
C. Date and time of incident
D. Actions taken

Q510. Which of the following storage practices is unsafe in a pharmacy setting?
A. Separating internal and external products
B. Storing insulin next to room-temperature medications
C. Labeling shelves by therapeutic class
D. Rotating inventory using FIFO
Q511. A technician notices a recurring pattern of wrong-dose errors during peak hours. What action supports CQI principles?
A. Ignore unless major harm occurs
B. Analyze workflow and staffing levels
C. Fire responsible employees
D. Reduce patient counseling time
Q512. Which abbreviation can be mistaken for "microgram"?
A. mcg
B. µg
C. mL
D. IU
Q513. What is the technician's role during an FDA drug recall?
A. Remove affected stock and quarantine it
B. Destroy all similar medications immediately
C. Notify prescribers personally
D. Dispense until new supply arrives
Q514. A technician receives a prescription for a medication the patient is allergic to. The correct action is to:
A. Fill the prescription and warn the patient
B. Hold the order and notify the pharmacist
C. Modify to an alternative drug
D. Delete the allergy note
Q515. Which practice supports error prevention in high-volume pharmacies?
A. Limiting communication among staff
B. Using bar-code verification and workflow queues
C. Assigning multiple tasks simultaneously
D. Ignoring automatic alerts
Q516. Which organization maintains national reporting programs for medication errors?
A. ISMP
B. CDC
C. DEA
D. OSHA
Q517. When cleaning counting trays used for antibiotics, which solution should be applied?
A. Sterile water
B. 70% isopropyl alcohol
C. Soap and cold water
D. Bleach
Q518. Which documentation detail is essential for a medication error report?
A. Staff opinions about causes
B. Exact product, lot, and expiration information
C. Pharmacy sales for the day
D. Approximate description of the event
Q519. Which pharmacy practice minimizes transcription errors?

A. Using verbal shortcuts
B. Entering all prescriptions immediately after receipt
C. Reading prescriptions twice before entry
D. Ignoring unclear handwriting

Q520. Which event requires an RCA (Root Cause Analysis)?
A. Expired drug pulled before use
B. Minor delay in prescription filling
C. Serious patient harm from a medication error
D. Typo corrected during verification

Q521. Which auxiliary label should appear on a reconstituted oral antibiotic like amoxicillin?
A. "Do not refrigerate"
B. "Shake well before use and refrigerate"
C. "Avoid sunlight"
D. "May cause drowsiness"

Q522. A technician encounters a spill of hazardous chemotherapy powder. What should be used first?
A. Paper towel
B. Spill kit and PPE
C. Regular gloves and cloth
D. Soap and water

Q523. A technician mislabels a medication as "20 mg" instead of "10 mg." What error type is this?
A. Wrong drug
B. Labeling error
C. Omission error
D. Dispensing error

Q524. What is the best preventive step against infection in sterile compounding areas?
A. Frequent surface cleaning and proper garbing
B. Allowing air recirculation from other rooms
C. Using scented lotions
D. Wearing nail polish

Q525. What is the technician's correct response to a pharmacy error identified by a patient?
A. Deny the error
B. Apologize, notify the pharmacist, and begin documentation
C. Offer a refund and no report
D. Blame another coworker

Q526. A technician discovers that a bottle of digoxin was stored without a desiccant packet. What should be done?
A. Dispense it anyway
B. Quarantine and inform the pharmacist
C. Add a new desiccant packet
D. Shake well before use

Q527. Which labeling instruction prevents overdose when dispensing oral liquids?
A. "Refrigerate after opening"
B. "Use calibrated dosing device provided"
C. "Avoid sunlight"
D. "Take on an empty stomach"

Q528. When compounding a sterile product, what action helps maintain first air to the critical site?
A. Placing hands behind the vial
B. Positioning objects to avoid airflow blockage

C. Resting supplies in front of the HEPA filter
D. Talking during manipulations

Q529. Which organization issues recommendations for preventing workplace exposure to hazardous drugs?
A. ISMP
B. NIOSH
C. DEA
D. USP

Q530. Which procedure minimizes risk when technicians prepare high-risk IV admixtures?
A. Performing calculation checks twice
B. Skipping final check due to experience
C. Using nonsterile gloves
D. Avoiding use of syringe filters

Q531. Which of the following should not be done when cleaning a biological safety cabinet?
A. Clean top to bottom, back to front
B. Use 70% isopropyl alcohol
C. Spray directly onto HEPA filter
D. Wipe horizontal surfaces methodically

Q532. A technician identifies a pattern of errors involving similar drug names. What should be the next step?
A. File individual incident reports only
B. Recommend Tall Man lettering and shelf separation
C. Ignore since pharmacist checks final products
D. Reduce lighting to avoid glare

Q533. A technician fails to record a refrigerator temperature for two consecutive days. What type of error is this?
A. Monitoring error
B. Documentation error
C. Omission error
D. Compliance error

Q534. Which abbreviation is unsafe because it may be confused with "morphine sulfate"?
A. MS
B. mg
C. mcg
D. mEq

Q535. When cleaning nonsterile compounding equipment, which step must be performed first?
A. Rinsing with alcohol
B. Removing visible residue with detergent and water
C. Spraying with disinfectant
D. Air drying immediately

Q536. What should a technician do if a patient reports nausea from a new medication?
A. Suggest taking with food
B. Refer to pharmacist for assessment
C. Advise stopping immediately
D. Tell them to ignore mild symptoms

Q537. A technician accidentally counts hydralazine instead of hydroxyzine. This is a:
A. LASA selection error
B. Documentation error

C. Omission error
D. Compliance error

Q538. Which PPE is mandatory when handling hazardous drug waste?
A. Hair cover only
B. Double chemotherapy gloves
C. Surgical mask only
D. No PPE needed

Q539. What is the technician's first action after discovering an unlabeled syringe in the compounding area?
A. Label it based on memory
B. Dispose of it immediately per policy
C. Ask another technician what it contains
D. Leave it until end of shift

Q540. A pharmacy technician must prepare an antibiotic suspension for a child. Which error prevention step is essential?
A. Verify with calibrated measuring tools
B. Estimate volume by eye
C. Skip reconstitution instructions
D. Mix powder directly in the stock bottle without verification

Q541. A patient reports that their medication label says "take 10 mg" but the doctor prescribed "1 mg." What is the error type?
A. Wrong drug
B. Labeling error
C. Wrong dose
D. Transcription error

Q542. What should be done with a controlled substance returned due to patient death?
A. Restock and reuse
B. Destroy following DEA and facility policy
C. Donate to charity
D. Ship directly to manufacturer

Q543. Which environmental monitoring test measures microbial contamination in cleanrooms?
A. Pressure differential
B. Air sampling
C. HEPA velocity test
D. Temperature log

Q544. What action should a technician take when a refrigerator alarm indicates a temperature deviation?
A. Reset alarm and ignore
B. Record temperature and notify the pharmacist
C. Adjust thermostat without logging
D. Continue operations normally

Q545. When preparing a chemotherapy IV, how should waste materials be disposed of?
A. Regular trash
B. Blue recycling container
C. Sharps bin for all materials
D. Yellow or trace chemotherapy waste container

Q546. Which term describes the proactive process of identifying risks before errors occur?
A. Root Cause Analysis (RCA)

B. Failure Mode and Effects Analysis (FMEA)
C. Continuous Quality Improvement (CQI)
D. Sentinel Event Reporting

Q547. A technician drops sterile gloves on the floor before use. What should they do?

A. Disinfect gloves and continue
B. Retrieve and reuse
C. Discard and replace with new sterile gloves
D. Continue compounding without gloves

Q548. A patient is dispensed prednisone instead of prednisolone. What type of error is this?

A. Wrong drug (LASA)
B. Wrong strength
C. Labeling
D. Documentation

Q549. Which of the following should be reported to OSHA?

A. Needle stick injury in compounding room
B. Expired stock discovered
C. Patient allergic reaction
D. Medication recall notice

Q550. A technician notices condensation inside the refrigerator storing vaccines. What should they do?

A. Ignore if temperatures appear normal
B. Document and notify pharmacist immediately
C. Adjust thermostat independently
D. Remove vaccines temporarily without record

Q551. Which element must always appear on a prescription label for outpatient dispensing?

A. Prescriber's DEA number
B. Pharmacy phone number
C. Patient's name
D. Lot number

Q552. A technician calculates the days' supply for a prescription written as "Take 1 tablet twice daily. Dispense 60 tablets." What is the correct days' supply?

A. 15 days
B. 30 days
C. 45 days
D. 60 days

Q553. What does the Sig code "1 cap po qid" mean?

A. One capsule by mouth twice daily
B. One capsule by mouth four times daily
C. One capsule by mouth every other day
D. One capsule by mouth three times daily

Q554. Which of the following is the correct formula for calculating total volume in a compounded prescription?

A. Quantity × Strength
B. Quantity ÷ Concentration
C. Dose ÷ Concentration
D. Volume × Time

Q555. What is the purpose of a National Drug Code (NDC)?

A. Identifies drug, manufacturer, and package size

B. Indicates expiration date
C. Tracks drug recall status only
D. Shows DEA classification

Q556. A medication order states "IVPB cefazolin 1 g q8h." What does "IVPB" mean?
A. Intravenous piggyback
B. Intravenous push bolus
C. Intramuscular injection
D. Infusion over 24 hours

Q557. When entering a prescription, the technician notices a dose twice the usual range. What should be done first?
A. Enter the prescription as written
B. Ask another technician for advice
C. Hold processing and notify the pharmacist
D. Call the prescriber directly

Q558. Which type of error is caused by choosing the wrong medication from a computer list during order entry?
A. Omission error
B. Wrong drug error
C. Monitoring error
D. Communication error

Q559. Which symbol indicates that a drug is a controlled substance under the Controlled Substances Act?
A. Rx only
B. C with Roman numeral inside
C. NDC
D. USP

Q560. Which of the following must be checked when returning medications to stock?
A. Patient insurance plan
B. NDC, lot number, and expiration date
C. Prescriber DEA number
D. Pharmacy license number

Q561. Which of the following describes "reverse distribution"?
A. Sending expired drugs to an authorized return processor
B. Repackaging bulk medication for dispensing
C. Disposing of sharps and hazardous waste
D. Returning medication to the patient

Q562. Which abbreviation should never appear on a prescription label?
A. BID
B. QHS
C. U
D. PO

Q563. Which of the following is required for a valid controlled prescription?
A. Patient's insurance ID
B. Prescriber's DEA number
C. Pharmacist's initials
D. Pharmacy NPI

Q564. What is the correct action when the prescriber omits the quantity to dispense?
A. Guess based on standard course

B. Contact prescriber for clarification
C. Dispense smallest stock bottle
D. Cancel the prescription

Q565. A technician receives a prescription for amoxicillin suspension requiring reconstitution. What must be verified before mixing?

A. Storage temperature
B. Prescriber's NPI
C. Correct diluent and final volume
D. Patient's insurance BIN

Q566. What type of prescription requires DEA Form 222 for ordering?

A. Schedule II
B. Schedule III
C. Schedule IV
D. Non-controlled

Q567. Which of the following is a key step in identifying expired medications in inventory?

A. Review lot numbers monthly
B. Use first-expire-first-out (FEFO) system
C. Recount all stock quarterly
D. Separate controlled substances

Q568. Which component of a prescription indicates how the patient should use the drug?

A. Inscription
B. Superscription
C. Subscription
D. Signa

Q569. What is the technician's next step if a written prescription appears to be altered?

A. Call the patient
B. Dispense a limited quantity
C. Notify the pharmacist immediately
D. Contact the DEA directly

Q570. Which step must a technician take after entering a new prescription before it's dispensed?

A. Give directly to patient
B. Have the pharmacist review and verify
C. Print label and apply immediately
D. File prescription for audit

Q571. Which of the following must appear on a controlled substance prescription label under federal law?

A. Pharmacy's phone number
B. Federal transfer warning
C. Prescriber's DEA registration certificate
D. NDC code

Q572. A patient's prescription reads "Take 2 tsp po bid." How many milliliters per day should be administered?

A. 10 mL
B. 15 mL
C. 20 mL
D. 40 mL

Q573. What should a technician do if a prescription's directions and quantity seem inconsistent?

A. Estimate a new quantity

B. Process it anyway
C. Hold for pharmacist clarification
D. Contact the insurance company

Q574. Which piece of information is required on all inpatient medication orders but not necessarily on outpatient prescriptions?
A. Patient date of birth
B. Room and bed number
C. Prescriber's DEA number
D. Patient address

Q575. Which of the following is an example of a calculation-based task in order entry?
A. Printing a prescription label
B. Determining day supply
C. Entering prescriber's name
D. Scanning a barcode

Q576. Which of the following drugs would most likely require refrigeration after reconstitution?
A. Amoxicillin suspension
B. Acetaminophen liquid
C. Loratadine syrup
D. Ibuprofen suspension

Q577. Which law requires tracking of controlled substances through the supply chain?
A. OBRA '90
B. Drug Supply Chain Security Act (DSCSA)
C. Controlled Substances Act (CSA)
D. Food, Drug, and Cosmetic Act (FDCA)

Q578. In the pharmacy computer system, which field identifies the prescriber uniquely?
A. DEA number
B. BIN number
C. NDC code
D. Rx number

Q579. What is the purpose of auxiliary labels?
A. Indicate medication name and strength
B. Provide additional usage or cautionary instructions
C. Replace the main prescription label
D. Show lot number for recall purposes

Q580. What information is required on a unit-dose package label for hospital use?
A. Patient name
B. Prescriber's signature
C. Expiration date and lot number
D. Billing code

Q581. Which of the following is true about DEA Form 41?
A. Used to order Schedule II drugs
B. Used to report theft of controlled substances
C. Used to document controlled substance destruction
D. Used to transfer controlled substances between pharmacies

Q582. What is the correct abbreviation for "before meals"?
A. QID
B. AC
C. PC

D. HS

Q583. A prescription label instructs "Take 1 tablet q12h for 10 days." How many tablets should be dispensed?

A. 10
B. 15
C. 20
D. 30

Q584. What is the correct first step when a controlled prescription appears altered?

A. Contact the prescriber to verify authenticity
B. Call the patient to confirm intent
C. Fill the prescription and document
D. Report immediately to local police

Q585. What device is commonly used to count tablets accurately in high-volume pharmacies?

A. Mortar and pestle
B. Automated tablet counter
C. Graduated cylinder
D. Compounding spatula

Q586. A patient's insurance rejects a refill too soon. What is the likely cause?

A. Expired prescription
B. Incorrect day supply entered
C. Invalid prescriber DEA
D. Incorrect NDC selection

Q587. A patient requests a transfer of a controlled prescription to another pharmacy. Which schedule may be transferred only once?

A. Schedule II
B. Schedule III
C. Schedule IV
D. Schedule V

Q588. What should be verified first when entering an e-prescription into the system?

A. Patient allergies
B. Insurance BIN number
C. Medication flavor preference
D. Pharmacy address

Q589. Which of the following actions best prevents look-alike/sound-alike drug errors?

A. Storing alphabetically
B. Using Tall Man lettering
C. Placing similar names together
D. Ignoring brand names

Q590. When entering a prescription, which field determines the reimbursement amount for the pharmacy?

A. NDC code
B. Rx number
C. BIN and PCN numbers
D. DEA number

Q591. When processing a refill request, what is the first item a technician should verify?

A. Insurance eligibility
B. Remaining refills authorized
C. Prescriber's address

D. Patient's phone number

Q592. Which of the following describes a key purpose of the lot number?

A. Identifies manufacturer and product for recall tracking
B. Determines billing price at point of sale
C. Indicates DEA classification
D. Verifies patient insurance coverage

Q593. What calculation determines the quantity of 250 mg tablets needed for a 10-day supply if the patient takes 500 mg twice daily?

A. 10
B. 20
C. 30
D. 40

Q594. Which information is NOT required on a prescription label under federal law?

A. Patient's name
B. Directions for use
C. Pharmacy address
D. Patient's insurance ID

Q595. Which of the following orders requires a pharmacist's verification of calculations before dispensing?

A. Amoxicillin 500 mg PO BID
B. Heparin 25,000 units in 500 mL IV infusion
C. Loratadine 10 mg PO daily
D. Acetaminophen 325 mg PO q4h PRN

Q596. Which form of error occurs when a technician enters "hydroxyzine" instead of "hydralazine"?

A. Wrong dose
B. Wrong drug
C. Wrong route
D. Omission

Q597. Which of the following must be recorded when returning a controlled substance to the supplier?

A. Prescriber's name
B. DEA Form 222
C. Pharmacy license number
D. Patient's ID

Q598. What abbreviation means "as needed"?

A. QD
B. HS
C. AC
D. PRN

Q599. What is the technician's most appropriate action when a patient reports an allergy during prescription entry?

A. Note it and proceed with filling
B. Enter it and alert the pharmacist
C. Ignore unless severe reaction
D. Ask patient to consult physician later

Q600. A label states "Take 1 tablet qid." How many hours apart should doses be taken?

A. Every 4 hours
B. Every 6 hours

C. Every 8 hours
D. Every 12 hours

Answer key and Explanation (501-600)

Q501. Answer: B

Explanation: Standardization—consistent labeling, forms, and workflows—reduces variability and human error. Skipping or ignoring verification introduces inconsistency. Memory-based processes lack reliability, especially in high-volume environments.

Q502. Answer: B

Explanation: Technicians participate in documentation and root-cause analysis (RCA) to identify workflow or procedural gaps. They cannot counsel or alter therapy. Their role supports system improvement through accurate factual reporting.

Q503. Answer: A

Explanation: Combining verbal and written pharmacist counseling reinforces comprehension, especially for complex regimens. Simplified, plain-language communication reduces misunderstanding. Labels alone often fail to ensure correct administration behavior.

Q504. Answer: B

Explanation: Cytotoxic or hazardous drug spills require full PPE, including a respirator mask, to prevent inhalation of aerosolized particles. Standard medication spills use gloves and gowns but not respirators. USP <800> defines these containment requirements.

Q505. Answer: A

Explanation: Unlabeled sterile preparations pose identification and contamination risks. Policy mandates immediate disposal to prevent accidental administration. Relabeling from memory or assumption endangers patients and violates USP <797> traceability standards.

Q506. Answer: B

Explanation: Warfarin is a high-alert medication because even small dosing errors can cause severe bleeding or clotting complications. ISMP classifies it as high risk. Amoxicillin, loratadine, and acetaminophen have wider safety margins and do not require such labeling.

Q507. Answer: A

Explanation: Skipping verification omits a critical safety step in the workflow, increasing risk of undetected errors. This is a process omission—failing to perform a required check. Wrong strength and wrong patient are specific outcomes, not the underlying cause.

Q508. Answer: B

Explanation: Jewelry and cosmetics shed particles and harbor microbes, increasing contamination risk. USP <797> prohibits them in cleanroom areas. Gloves alone cannot offset improper hygiene. Touching sterile parts or leaving supplies open also compromises asepsis.

Q509. Answer: B

Explanation: Documentation must remain factual, including times, details, and corrective actions. Emotional or subjective wording introduces bias and undermines clarity. Objective records are vital for CQI review and regulatory compliance.

Q510. Answer: B

Explanation: Insulin requires refrigeration; storing it beside room-temperature medications risks potency loss. Temperature-sensitive products must remain in controlled environments. FIFO rotation and clear labeling support accuracy and compliance.

Q511. Answer: B

Explanation: CQI emphasizes system-based improvement, not punishment. Analyzing workflow, workload, and staffing identifies root causes. Adjustments to procedures, not discipline, drive sustainable error reduction. Ignoring trends contradicts safety culture values.

Q512. Answer: B

Explanation: The symbol "µg" is easily confused with "mg," causing 1000-fold dosing errors. Writing "mcg" in full prevents confusion. ISMP and Joint Commission both recommend avoiding "µg" in any written or electronic order.

Q513. Answer: A

Explanation: Technicians must identify, segregate, and quarantine recalled medications under pharmacist supervision. Destruction or dispensing continues only after official instructions. Proper recordkeeping ensures compliance and traceability during the recall process.

Q514. Answer: B

Explanation: Technicians must stop the process and alert the pharmacist, who will contact the prescriber for alternatives. Filling or altering the order independently is outside the technician's scope and risks patient harm.

Q515. Answer: B

Explanation: Bar-code verification and structured workflow queues automate safety checks and prevent distractions during multitasking. Open communication enhances vigilance. Ignoring alerts or multitasking increases cognitive overload and error risk.

Q516. Answer: A

Explanation: The Institute for Safe Medication Practices (ISMP) collects voluntary error reports and analyzes national trends to improve safety. DEA manages controlled substances, CDC handles disease control, and OSHA enforces workplace safety—not medication error reporting.

Q517. Answer: B

Explanation: 70% isopropyl alcohol effectively disinfects counting trays and evaporates without residue. It kills most microorganisms and prevents cross-contamination. Soap, bleach, or water may leave residues or damage the tray's surface.

Q518. Answer: B

Explanation: Complete product identification, including lot and expiration data, enables tracking and recall linkage. Approximate or opinion-based entries lack legal and analytical value. Accurate, factual reporting is mandatory in CQI documentation.

Q519. Answer: C

Explanation: Double-reading ensures comprehension and accuracy before entry. Clarifying ambiguous orders with the pharmacist avoids dangerous transcription errors. Ignoring or assuming unclear handwriting violates safety protocols.

Q520. Answer: C

Explanation: RCA is performed after severe harm or sentinel events to identify underlying process failures. Routine corrections or delays don't warrant RCA. This analysis helps prevent recurrence through systemic improvement.

Q521. Answer: B

Explanation: Many reconstituted antibiotics require refrigeration to maintain stability and must be shaken to evenly disperse particles. "Shake well and refrigerate" ensures therapeutic effectiveness. Other labels apply to unrelated medications.

Q522. Answer: B

Explanation: Hazardous drug spills must be handled immediately using a designated spill kit and appropriate PPE per USP <800>. Paper towels and regular gloves offer inadequate protection and risk contamination or inhalation.

Q523. Answer: B

Explanation: Incorrect labeling of the correct drug strength is a labeling error. Dispensing or wrong-drug errors involve incorrect product selection. Label accuracy is essential to patient safety and compliance.

Q524. Answer: A

Explanation: USP <797> mandates regular cleaning with sterile disinfectants and full garbing to minimize contamination. Lotions and cosmetics compromise glove integrity and should be avoided. Controlled airflow maintains asepsis.

Q525. Answer: B

Explanation: The technician should acknowledge the patient's concern, notify the pharmacist immediately, and help document the event. Transparency and prompt action uphold ethical standards and facilitate corrective procedures without blame.

Q526. Answer: B

Explanation: Moisture-sensitive medications like digoxin require desiccants to maintain stability. Missing desiccants compromise drug potency. Quarantine and pharmacist review ensure evaluation before use or disposal. Adding desiccant after exposure doesn't restore integrity.

Q527. Answer: B

Explanation: Instructing patients to use a calibrated dosing device ensures accurate measurement, preventing under- or overdosing. Household spoons cause dosing variability. Other labels relate to storage or absorption, not dose accuracy.

Q528. Answer: B

Explanation: Maintaining unobstructed airflow (first air) between HEPA filter and critical site prevents microbial contamination. Placing hands or objects in front of the airflow interrupts this protective barrier, compromising sterility.

Q529. Answer: B

Explanation: The National Institute for Occupational Safety and Health (NIOSH) provides detailed guidance on handling hazardous drugs safely. USP enforces compounding standards, while ISMP and DEA focus on error prevention and controlled substances, respectively.

Q530. Answer: A

Explanation: Independent double verification of all calculations and ingredients ensures accuracy for high-risk sterile products. Skipping checks or using improper PPE invites contamination or dosing errors. Verification is required by USP <797> for all compounded sterile preparations.

Q531. Answer: C

Explanation: HEPA filters must never be sprayed directly because moisture damages filter fibers and airflow integrity. Cleaning should focus on surfaces using lint-free wipes and alcohol. Proper order prevents recontamination and preserves sterile conditions.

Q532. Answer: B

Explanation: Tall Man lettering and physical separation of LASA drugs reduce confusion and are proven ISMP strategies. Reporting alone without system changes doesn't solve recurring issues. Adequate lighting enhances visibility and accuracy.

Q533. Answer: B

Explanation: Missing required documentation—like temperature logs—constitutes a documentation error. Monitoring errors relate to unrecognized therapy outcomes, while omission errors refer to missed doses. Documentation lapses affect audit compliance and quality assurance integrity.

Q534. Answer: A

Explanation: "MS" can mean either morphine sulfate or magnesium sulfate, leading to potentially fatal misinterpretations. Always write the full drug name. ISMP classifies this abbreviation as high risk.

Q535. Answer: B

Explanation: Cleaning begins with removal of visible residues using detergent and water to eliminate gross contamination. Disinfection follows. Skipping detergent cleaning leaves residues that interfere with disinfectants and product integrity.

Q536. Answer: B

Explanation: Technicians must refer all adverse reaction reports to the pharmacist, who can assess severity and contact the prescriber if needed. Providing medical advice exceeds technician scope and could harm the patient.

Q537. Answer: A

Explanation: Hydralazine and hydroxyzine are classic LASA drugs. Selecting one instead of the other represents a LASA selection error. This highlights the importance of Tall Man lettering and barcode scanning for verification.

Q538. Answer: B

Explanation: Double gloves specifically tested for chemotherapy agents protect against dermal exposure during handling or disposal. Single gloves or masks are insufficient per USP <800>. Proper PPE ensures worker safety.

Q539. Answer: B

Explanation: Unlabeled syringes present a major safety hazard. They must be discarded immediately according to facility policy. Reusing or guessing contents violates sterile compounding standards and could cause fatal errors.

Q540. Answer: A

Explanation: Using calibrated devices ensures accuracy in water volume and concentration during reconstitution. Estimation or skipping verification leads to incorrect dosing. Proper measurement guarantees therapeutic safety and efficacy.

Q541. Answer: C

Explanation: Dispensing 10 mg instead of 1 mg is a wrong dose error that could lead to overdose. This usually occurs during transcription or labeling stages. Final pharmacist verification helps intercept such mistakes.

Q542. Answer: B

Explanation: Controlled substances must be destroyed per DEA regulations, witnessed by authorized personnel. Restocking or donation violates law. Documentation of destruction ensures compliance and accountability.

Q543. Answer: B

Explanation: Air sampling evaluates microbial levels in compounding areas to verify sterile conditions. Pressure and velocity measure airflow dynamics, while temperature logging tracks environmental stability. Airborne particle control ensures product safety.

Q544. Answer: B

Explanation: Documenting deviations and alerting the pharmacist ensures assessment of medication stability. Silent resets obscure data needed for compliance and corrective action. Immediate reporting protects product potency and regulatory adherence.

Q545. Answer: D

Explanation: Chemotherapy-related waste, including tubing and PPE, must go into designated yellow trace chemotherapy containers per USP <800>. Regular trash or sharps bins are inappropriate for hazardous materials.

Q546. Answer: B

Explanation: FMEA is a proactive process that predicts potential failure points in a system to prevent future errors. RCA is reactive, performed after events. CQI focuses on long-term improvement, while sentinel event reporting follows major incidents.

Q547. Answer: C

Explanation: Once gloves contact non-sterile surfaces, sterility is compromised. They must be replaced immediately to maintain aseptic conditions. Disinfection cannot restore sterility for dropped gloves. Proper glove management prevents contamination.

Q548. Answer: A

Explanation: Prednisone and prednisolone are classic LASA drugs that differ in potency and formulation. Dispensing the wrong one is a LASA-related wrong drug error. Proper barcode scanning and Tall Man lettering help prevent mix-ups.

Q549. Answer: A

Explanation: Occupational exposure incidents, such as needle sticks or hazardous material spills, must be reported to OSHA under workplace safety rules. Patient-specific reactions and recalls fall under FDA or facility reporting systems.

Q550. Answer: B

Explanation: Condensation may signal temperature instability or seal failure. Documentation and immediate pharmacist notification ensure vaccines are assessed for potency. Independent adjustment without record breaches compliance and traceability.

Q551. Answer: C

Explanation: The patient's name is required on every outpatient prescription label to ensure proper identification and prevent dispensing errors. Although the pharmacy phone number and DEA number may appear, they are not mandatory in all jurisdictions. The lot number is used internally for recalls and tracking, not typically printed on outpatient labels.

Q552. Answer: B

Explanation: Two tablets are taken each day (1 tablet BID), so 60 ÷ 2 = 30 days. The nearest distractor, 60 days, ignores dosing frequency. Incorrectly calculating the days' supply may cause billing or refill errors, so verifying dosage frequency against quantity dispensed is essential in order entry accuracy.

Q553. Answer: B

Explanation: "po" means by mouth, and "qid" means four times daily. This Sig directs oral administration of one capsule four times per day. The distractor "tid" (three times daily) is often confused with "qid." Reading Sig codes carefully ensures proper patient labeling and prevents dosing frequency errors during order entry.

Q554. Answer: C

Explanation: The formula for finding volume needed is Dose ÷ Concentration. For example, 250 mg ÷ (125 mg/mL) = 2 mL. Distractors such as "Quantity × Strength" confuse amount and concentration relationships. Accurate conversions prevent underdosing or overdosing during compounding and order entry.

Q555. Answer: A

Explanation: The NDC uniquely identifies the product: first segment = manufacturer, second = drug and strength, third = package size. Distractors like expiration date or DEA class are unrelated. Using the correct NDC ensures accuracy during drug selection, billing, and inventory control in the order entry process.

Q556. Answer: A

Explanation: "IVPB" refers to an intravenous piggyback—a secondary infusion attached to a primary line. The distractor "IV push" is faster and involves direct injection. Understanding abbreviations like IVPB prevents route errors and ensures appropriate administration timing in the medication order process.

Q557. Answer: C

Explanation: The technician must always alert the pharmacist when a dose seems inappropriate before processing. Only the pharmacist may contact the prescriber for clarification. Distractors such as entering it or consulting another technician violate patient safety protocols and workflow responsibilities in order entry.

Q558. Answer: B

Explanation: Selecting an incorrect medication during entry is a wrong drug error. Omission errors involve skipped doses, and communication errors involve misinterpretation. Double-checking drug name, strength, and NDC helps prevent sound-alike/look-alike medication mix-ups common in computerized systems.

Q559. Answer: B

Explanation: A capital "C" with a Roman numeral (I–V) denotes the schedule of a controlled substance. "Rx only" means prescription-only, not controlled. The NDC identifies the drug, while "USP" refers to quality standards. Recognizing control symbols helps technicians manage storage, ordering, and documentation correctly.

Q560. Answer: B

Explanation: When restocking medications, verifying the NDC, lot number, and expiration date ensures product integrity and traceability. DEA or license numbers are not relevant here. Returning wrong-lot medications may complicate recalls or cause patient safety issues, so accurate verification is crucial.

Q561. Answer: A

Explanation: Reverse distribution involves returning expired or recalled drugs to an authorized handler for credit or disposal. It differs from repackaging, which is for internal use. The process helps maintain compliance with federal waste management laws and ensures safe removal of unusable products from inventory.

Q562. Answer: C

Explanation: The abbreviation "U" for "units" is unsafe—it may be mistaken as a zero. The other terms (BID, QHS, PO) are standard when interpreted properly. Avoiding dangerous abbreviations follows ISMP and Joint Commission guidelines for medication safety and error prevention during labeling.

Q563. Answer: B

Explanation: The prescriber's DEA number is legally required on all controlled substance prescriptions. Pharmacist initials confirm verification, not prescription validity. Insurance ID and pharmacy NPI are administrative. Missing DEA numbers make controlled scripts non-compliant.

Q564. Answer: B

Explanation: Only the prescriber can authorize quantity; technicians or pharmacists cannot assume or estimate. Contacting the prescriber ensures accuracy and legal compliance. Dispensing without clarification violates pharmacy regulations and patient safety standards. Documentation of the clarification is also required.

Q565. Answer: C

Explanation: Before reconstitution, confirm the diluent type and amount to reach the proper final volume. Wrong diluent or miscalculated volume affects concentration and dosing accuracy. While storage and NPI are important later, they do not ensure correct preparation.

Q566. Answer: A

Explanation: DEA Form 222 is mandatory for ordering Schedule II controlled substances. Schedules III–V require standard invoices instead. Failure to use Form 222 may result in DEA violations. The form tracks controlled drugs through the supply chain for accountability and diversion prevention.

Q567. Answer: B

Explanation: The FEFO method ensures the earliest expiration dates are dispensed first, minimizing waste and avoiding dispensing expired products. While lot review and inventory counts support this, FEFO is the most direct expiration control system. Controlled substance segregation addresses security, not expiration tracking.

Q568. Answer: D

Explanation: The Signa (Sig) gives patient directions—dose, route, frequency, and timing. The inscription lists ingredients, the superscription is "Rx," and the subscription provides compounding instructions. Proper interpretation of the Signa ensures accurate labeling and patient adherence in order entry.

Q569. Answer: C

Explanation: Technicians must notify the pharmacist immediately about any suspected forgery or alteration. Only the pharmacist or DEA can investigate further. Dispensing any portion violates law. Prompt reporting protects the pharmacy from legal risk and prevents diversion.

Q570. Answer: B

Explanation: Every new prescription entry must undergo pharmacist verification before dispensing to ensure safety and accuracy. Printing or handing medication before review violates pharmacy law and safety protocols. The pharmacist is responsible for final clinical and legal verification before release.

Q571. Answer: B

Explanation: Controlled substance labels must include the federal transfer warning: "Caution: Federal law prohibits the transfer of this drug to any person other than the patient..." The DEA certificate is not printed on the label. NDC codes are used internally, and the phone number is optional. This warning prevents diversion and misuse.

Q572. Answer: C

Explanation: One teaspoon equals 5 mL. The order is 2 tsp (10 mL) twice daily, for a total of 20 mL daily. The distractor 10 mL reflects one dose, not daily intake. Accurate conversions between household and metric units are essential to prevent dosing errors in dispensing.

Q573. Answer: C

Explanation: When any inconsistency exists between directions and quantity, the technician must hold the prescription for pharmacist review. Only a pharmacist may clarify with the prescriber. Estimating or altering the order risks safety violations and billing errors. Always prioritize accuracy and legal compliance in processing.

Q574. Answer: B

Explanation: Room and bed numbers are used for inpatient medication administration tracking but are not required for outpatient scripts. Patient address and prescriber DEA numbers apply mainly to outpatient controlled prescriptions. Correctly identifying inpatient locations ensures proper delivery and avoids administration mix-ups.

Q575. Answer: B

Explanation: Day-supply determination requires mathematical calculation based on dose frequency and quantity. It affects insurance billing, refill timing, and inventory control. The other tasks—printing, entering, and scanning—are administrative and require accuracy but not computation. Calculating days' supply ensures compliance with payer and clinical standards.

Q576. Answer: A

Explanation: Amoxicillin suspension requires refrigeration after reconstitution to maintain stability and potency. The others—acetaminophen, loratadine, ibuprofen—are commercially prepared liquids that remain stable at room temperature. Proper storage labeling is essential to maintain medication integrity and ensure accurate patient counseling.

Q577. Answer: B

Explanation: The DSCSA mandates tracing prescription drug products through the supply chain to prevent counterfeit distribution. The CSA governs controlled substance scheduling, while OBRA '90 relates to counseling and drug use review. Understanding federal acts ensures compliance in order tracking and record-keeping.

Q578. Answer: A

Explanation: A DEA number uniquely identifies prescribers authorized to issue controlled prescriptions. BIN numbers route insurance claims, NDC codes describe drugs, and Rx numbers identify prescriptions. Verifying DEA information ensures legal prescribing and helps detect fraudulent or forged prescriptions during entry.

Q579. Answer: B

Explanation: Auxiliary labels communicate supplementary information like "Take with food" or "May cause drowsiness." They reinforce patient understanding but do not replace main labels. Including them correctly helps reduce medication misuse and supports patient safety in the dispensing process.

Q580. Answer: C

Explanation: Each unit-dose package must list the drug name, strength, expiration date, and lot number for traceability. Patient name and prescriber information are not included since doses are assigned later. Correct labeling ensures safe administration and recall management in institutional settings.

Q581. Answer: C

Explanation: DEA Form 41 documents destruction of controlled substances. DEA Form 222 is for ordering, Form 106 for theft or loss, and transfers require special invoices. Proper documentation of disposal prevents diversion and maintains DEA compliance in pharmacy operations.

Q582. Answer: B

Explanation: "AC" stands for ante cibum, meaning before meals. "PC" means after meals, "HS" means at bedtime, and "QID" is four times daily. Knowing Latin abbreviations ensures proper interpretation of medication directions and accurate label generation during order entry.

Q583. Answer: C

Explanation: Every 12 hours equals two doses daily. Over 10 days: $2 \times 10 = 20$ tablets. Misinterpreting frequency could underdose or overdose the patient. Double-checking Sig math prevents refill and therapy duration errors during prescription processing.

Q584. Answer: A

Explanation: If alteration is suspected, the pharmacist must verify with the prescriber before dispensing. Filling or reporting immediately without verification can breach procedure. Once confirmed fraudulent, the pharmacy should then notify DEA or authorities per policy.

Q585. Answer: B

Explanation: Automated tablet counters improve efficiency and reduce human error in counting solid dosage forms. Mortar and pestle or spatula are used for compounding, not counting. Graduated cylinders measure liquids. Automation enhances accuracy and productivity in order processing.

Q586. Answer: B

Explanation: Insurance systems compare refill timing to the entered day supply. Entering it incorrectly (too short) triggers "refill too soon." The other issues—expired script or wrong NDC—cause different rejections. Correct day-supply entry ensures smooth claim processing and compliance.

Q587. Answer: C

Explanation: Schedules III–V may be transferred once between pharmacies, except electronically shared real-time systems. Schedule II cannot be transferred at all. Understanding transfer restrictions prevents legal violations and ensures controlled substance accountability.

Q588. Answer: A

Explanation: Allergies must always be verified first to prevent adverse reactions. Insurance and address can be corrected later, but an allergy mismatch could result in serious harm. Allergy checks are a vital safety step in every order entry process.

Q589. Answer: B

Explanation: Tall Man lettering (e.g., hydrOXYzine vs. hydrALAzine) visually differentiates similar drug names, reducing selection errors. Alphabetical storage can increase confusion, while grouping look-alike drugs together worsens risk. Implementing ISMP-recommended Tall Man strategies enhances safety in order entry.

Q590. Answer: A

Explanation: The NDC code identifies the specific product dispensed, which directly determines reimbursement. BIN and PCN route claims, but NDC defines cost. Accurate NDC selection ensures correct billing and prevents audit discrepancies in the order entry process.

Q591. Answer: B
Explanation: The technician must first confirm that authorized refills remain on the prescription before processing. Filling without authorization violates federal and state laws. Insurance or contact details can be verified afterward. Confirming refills ensures compliance and prevents dispensing beyond the prescriber's intent.
Q592. Answer: A
Explanation: The lot number tracks drug batches for recall or quality issues. It links each dispensed product to its manufacturing source. Pricing, DEA schedule, or insurance are unrelated. Maintaining lot traceability supports safety and regulatory compliance during order entry and dispensing.
Q593. Answer: D
Explanation: Each dose is 500 mg, which equals two 250 mg tablets. Two doses per day for 10 days = 2 × 2 × 10 = 40 tablets. Confusing strength versus dosage would lead to underdosing. Proper conversion ensures accurate quantity during processing.
Q594. Answer: D
Explanation: Insurance ID is not part of the legal prescription label requirements. The label must show patient name, prescriber, drug name, directions, pharmacy details, and fill date. Including unnecessary identifiers may violate privacy without adding clinical value.
Q595. Answer: B
Explanation: Heparin IV infusions require pharmacist verification because they involve complex dosage and dilution calculations. Routine oral medications like loratadine or acetaminophen use standard doses. Calculation-based parenteral orders demand double-checking to prevent life-threatening dosing errors.
Q596. Answer: B
Explanation: Selecting hydroxyzine instead of hydralazine is a wrong drug error, often due to look-alike/sound-alike confusion. Wrong dose or route errors involve the correct medication but incorrect parameters. Verifying NDC and drug class prevents these substitution mistakes during data entry.
Q597. Answer: B
Explanation: A DEA Form 222 must accompany all returns of Schedule II controlled substances. It documents product, quantity, and transaction details. Pharmacy license or prescriber data are not required for this step. Maintaining complete DEA records ensures compliance and prevents diversion.
Q598. Answer: D
Explanation: PRN stands for "pro re nata," meaning as needed. QD means once daily, AC means before meals, and HS means at bedtime. Understanding Latin abbreviations helps ensure accurate patient labeling and counseling in pharmacy practice.
Q599. Answer: B
Explanation: The technician should document the allergy in the system and alert the pharmacist immediately. Only the pharmacist evaluates clinical significance. Ignoring or delaying this step could cause adverse reactions. Allergy documentation is critical for patient safety in every dispensing process.
Q600. Answer: B
Explanation: "QID" means four times daily, which corresponds to approximately every 6 hours (24 ÷ 4 = 6). Confusing it with every 4 hours (which would be six times daily) can cause overdosing. Understanding dosing intervals ensures accurate timing and compliance.

Questions (601-650)

Q601. What is the purpose of verifying the NDC number during order entry?

A. Confirms the patient's address

B. Ensures drug, manufacturer, and strength match the order

C. Displays insurance pricing

D. Confirms prescriber authority

Q602. What document is used to record details of a prescription error or near miss?

A. Controlled Substance Log

B. Medication Administration Record

C. DEA Form 106

D. Quality Assurance Report

Q603. Which of the following must be verified before processing an insurance claim?

A. Prescriber's DEA number

B. Patient's date of birth

C. Pharmacy's NPI

D. Manufacturer's lot number

Q604. What is the usual route of administration for insulin?

A. Oral

B. Subcutaneous

C. Intravenous

D. Intramuscular

Q605. Which type of prescription requires tamper-resistant paper under federal law?

A. Over-the-counter

B. Veterinary medications

C. Non-controlled maintenance drugs

D. Controlled substances

Q606. What step should follow printing a prescription label?

A. Immediate patient handoff

B. Pharmacist verification of contents

C. Filing the hard copy

D. Billing submission

Q607. Which calculation is used to find the total mL dispensed if 5 mL is given q6h for 7 days?

A. 140 mL

B. 120 mL

C. 100 mL

D. 80 mL

Q608. Which of the following helps prevent medication selection errors on automated dispensing screens?

A. Ignoring NDC codes

B. Disabling tall man lettering

C. Verifying drug name, strength, and dosage form before selection

D. Speeding through data entry

Q609. Which of the following is an example of a data entry error?

A. Entering incorrect quantity

B. Printing a duplicate label

C. Counting pills inaccurately

D. Placing the wrong cap on a bottle

Q610. Which field in a pharmacy system tracks each medication dispensed for a patient over time?
A. Drug Utilization Review (DUR) log
B. Patient profile
C. Inventory report
D. Controlled substance log
Q611. A prescription reads "2 gtt ou qid." What does this mean?
A. Two drops in both eyes four times daily
B. Two drops in right eye four times daily
C. Two drops in left ear four times daily
D. Two drops in both ears every other day
Q612. What does "QS ad 100 mL" mean on a compounding formula?
A. Add sufficient quantity to make 100 mL total volume
B. Add 100 mL of active ingredient
C. Add 100 mL of diluent
D. Dispense 100 mL extra
Q613. What is the most appropriate action if a technician notices a missing DEA number on a Schedule II prescription?
A. Process it anyway
B. Add a known DEA number manually
C. Alert the pharmacist for verification
D. Call insurance for override
Q614. What label warning is mandatory for all controlled substance prescriptions?
A. For external use only
B. May cause drowsiness
C. Federal transfer caution
D. Take with food
Q615. Which part of a prescription authorizes the pharmacist to prepare the medication?
A. Superscription
B. Subscription
C. Signa
D. Inscription
Q616. When calculating the final concentration of a reconstituted medication, which information is essential?
A. NDC code and expiration date
B. Manufacturer name and DEA schedule
C. Powder strength and diluent volume
D. Patient name and storage temperature
Q617. Which of the following medications would most likely require a filter needle for preparation?
A. Ampicillin injection
B. Lidocaine vial
C. Glass ampule medication
D. Insulin suspension
Q618. What is the correct meaning of the abbreviation "NPO"?
A. Take with food
B. Nothing by mouth
C. Take as needed
D. Do not crush

Q619. When entering an electronic prescription, which field must be double-checked to prevent wrong-patient errors?
A. Patient name and date of birth
B. BIN number
C. Prescriber DEA
D. Pharmacy NPI
Q620. Which type of label includes the drug name, strength, lot number, and expiration date but not patient information?
A. Stock bottle label
B. Unit-dose label
C. Prescription label
D. Auxiliary label
Q621. How many milligrams of drug are in 30 mL of a 250 mg/5 mL solution?
A. 1000 mg
B. 1250 mg
C. 1500 mg
D. 2500 mg
Q622. What is the proper action if a controlled substance shipment arrives missing one bottle?
A. Record shortage on DEA Form 106
B. Contact prescriber for replacement
C. Reorder next month
D. Ignore if partial box arrived
Q623. Which of the following represents a correct pharmacy calculation formula?
A. Desired ÷ Have × Quantity
B. Have ÷ Desired × Quantity
C. Quantity ÷ Have × Desired
D. Desired × Have ÷ Quantity
Q624. Which of the following prescriptions should be clarified due to missing directions?
A. Lisinopril 10 mg tablet #30
B. Amoxicillin 500 mg cap TID for 10 days
C. Metformin 500 mg BID with meals
D. Atorvastatin 20 mg daily
Q625. Which auxiliary label should accompany an antibiotic suspension?
A. Take with milk
B. Keep refrigerated, shake well before use
C. May cause dizziness
D. Take on an empty stomach
Q626. A prescription is written for "metoprolol 50 mg PO BID." What is the total daily dose?
A. 50 mg
B. 75 mg
C. 100 mg
D. 150 mg
Q627. Which of the following tasks is within a technician's scope during order entry?
A. Counseling the patient
B. Calling the prescriber to change therapy
C. Entering patient and prescription information accurately
D. Approving therapeutic substitutions
Q628. What is the correct meaning of the abbreviation "TID"?

A. Every 4 hours
B. Three times daily
C. Twice daily
D. Every other day

Q629. What must be done if the computer system flags a potential drug–drug interaction?
A. Override the warning and continue
B. Ignore unless the patient complains
C. Notify the pharmacist for evaluation
D. Ask another technician for advice

Q630. Which of the following actions ensures accurate counting of tablets?
A. Counting directly by hand
B. Using a calibrated counting tray and spatula
C. Estimating quantity visually
D. Using paper to scoop tablets

Q631. What is the primary purpose of the SIG line on a prescription label?
A. Display drug expiration date
B. Provide prescriber's instructions to the patient
C. Record insurance claim details
D. Identify manufacturer

Q632. Which of the following represents a correct example of a metric conversion?
A. 1 teaspoon = 10 mL
B. 1 tablespoon = 15 mL
C. 1 ounce = 20 mL
D. 1 pint = 300 mL

Q633. Which reference is most appropriate to verify the correct spelling of a drug name during entry?
A. DEA Manual
B. FDA Recall Database
C. Drug Facts and Comparisons
D. Manufacturer's invoice

Q634. What is the technician's responsibility when the computer system shows duplicate therapy alerts?
A. Delete one of the medications
B. Notify the pharmacist for review
C. Proceed with the newer order only
D. Ask the patient which to keep

Q635. When entering a new prescription, which information should be double-checked to prevent insurance claim denial?
A. BIN, PCN, and ID numbers
B. NDC code only
C. Prescriber's address
D. Patient's allergy list

Q636. Which of the following must appear on a compounded medication label?
A. Patient diagnosis
B. Beyond-use date
C. Prescriber's DEA number
D. Manufacturer lot number

Q637. Which controlled substance schedule cannot be refilled under any circumstance?
A. Schedule II

B. Schedule III
C. Schedule IV
D. Schedule V

Q638. When performing dosage calculations, what should the technician do if the result seems unusually high?

A. Round up to the nearest whole tablet
B. Continue since it matches the written order
C. Stop and alert the pharmacist immediately
D. Reduce by half automatically

Q639. What does the acronym "DAW" on a prescription stand for?

A. Dispense as written
B. Drug and warning
C. Dosage and weight
D. Dispense at will

Q640. A 500 mL IV bag is to infuse at 125 mL/hour. How long will the infusion last?

A. 2 hours
B. 3 hours
C. 4 hours
D. 5 hours

Q641. What is the correct action if a prescription's directions are illegible?

A. Guess based on prior prescriptions
B. Ask another technician
C. Have the pharmacist contact the prescriber
D. Skip directions on the label

Q642. Which of the following tasks should a technician perform when restocking medications?

A. Record lot numbers and expiration dates
B. Repackage controlled substances
C. Change beyond-use dates
D. Alter manufacturer labeling

Q643. Which component of a prescription contains the drug name and strength?

A. Inscription
B. Superscription
C. Subscription
D. Signa

Q644. Which of the following is true regarding the handling of expired medications?

A. May be dispensed until replaced
B. Must be quarantined and separated from active stock
C. Can be restocked if unopened
D. Can be donated to another pharmacy

Q645. Which type of order is commonly used for a single administration in hospitals?

A. Standing order
B. PRN order
C. STAT order
D. Routine order

Q646. When calculating total daily dose for "morphine 10 mg IV q4h," what is the total amount administered in 24 hours?

A. 40 mg
B. 50 mg

C. 60 mg
D. 70 mg

Q647. What is the key purpose of a final pharmacist check before dispensing?
A. Print the patient receipt
B. Verify accuracy, legality, and appropriateness of the prescription
C. Approve technician work hours
D. Submit the insurance claim

Q648. Which of the following actions best helps prevent transcription errors during prescription entry?
A. Skipping duplicate checks to save time
B. Reading back and verifying entries with the original order
C. Relying on auto-fill features in the computer
D. Entering multiple prescriptions simultaneously

Q649. What is the correct meaning of the abbreviation "PC"?
A. After meals
B. Before meals
C. At bedtime
D. As needed

Q650. A prescription reads: "Amoxicillin 250 mg/5 mL, take 10 mL PO TID for 10 days." How many milliliters are needed to fill this order?
A. 150 mL
B. 200 mL
C. 250 mL
D. 300 mL

Answer key and Explanation (601-650)

Q601. Answer: B

Explanation: The NDC number confirms the exact drug product, strength, and manufacturer. Using the wrong NDC may result in incorrect medication or billing errors. It's unrelated to address, pricing, or prescriber credentials. Verification prevents product mismatches during dispensing.

Q602. Answer: C

Explanation: A Quality Assurance Report records prescription errors and near misses to analyze and prevent future incidents. DEA Form 106 documents theft or loss, not errors. Reporting and reviewing these events improve safety and compliance through continuous quality improvement.

Q603. Answer: B

Explanation: Insurance claims require accurate patient identifiers, especially date of birth, to match profiles. DEA and NPI numbers identify professionals, not patients. Lot numbers are unrelated to billing. Incorrect demographic data leads to claim rejections and processing delays.

Q604. Answer: B

Explanation: Insulin is administered subcutaneously for gradual absorption. IV or IM routes are used only in emergencies by healthcare providers. Oral insulin is not effective because digestive enzymes degrade it. Recognizing proper routes prevents entry and labeling errors in prescriptions.

Q605. Answer: D

Explanation: Controlled substances must be written on tamper-resistant paper to prevent alteration or forgery. Non-controlled or OTC drugs are not federally required to use it, though some states extend the rule. Ensuring proper paper use supports regulatory and legal compliance.

Q606. Answer: B

Explanation: After label printing, pharmacist verification ensures that medication, strength, directions, and patient match the original order. Dispensing prior to verification is illegal and unsafe. Verification is the final safety checkpoint before release.

Q607. Answer: A

Explanation: $24 \div 6 = 4$ doses/day $\times$ 7 days = 28 doses. 28×5 mL = 140 mL total. Miscalculating frequency leads to incorrect quantity, affecting refill timing. Accurate computation ensures proper therapy duration and billing precision.

Q608. Answer: C

Explanation: Verifying drug name, strength, and dosage form prevents wrong-drug selection on electronic systems. Ignoring NDCs or Tall Man lettering increases confusion. Accuracy, not speed, ensures patient safety. Careful screen review reduces sound-alike/look-alike errors during the order entry process.

Q609. Answer: A

Explanation: Entering an incorrect quantity is a data entry error that occurs during transcription in the computer system. The others—counting or labeling issues—are dispensing errors. Proper data verification ensures prescription accuracy before filling or billing begins.

Q610. Answer: B

Explanation: The patient profile stores the complete medication history, including allergies, active prescriptions, and refill data. DUR uses this profile to identify interactions. Inventory and controlled substance logs serve operational purposes, not patient-specific tracking.

Q611. Answer: A

Explanation: "Gtt" = drops, "ou" = both eyes, and "qid" = four times daily. Therefore, two drops in both eyes four times per day. Misreading ocular/otic abbreviations can cause wrong-site administration. Knowing common Latin abbreviations ensures proper interpretation.

Q612. Answer: A

Explanation: "QS ad" means quantity sufficient to make a specified total. Thus, add enough base to reach 100 mL. The distractors misunderstand "QS" as a fixed addition. Precise volume adjustments ensure accurate concentration in compounded preparations.

Q613. Answer: C

Explanation: Only a pharmacist can verify or obtain a missing DEA number from the prescriber. Technicians cannot enter or alter this legally required information. Filling without verification violates DEA rules. Proper escalation maintains compliance and accountability.

Q614. Answer: C

Explanation: Controlled substance labels must bear the federal transfer warning: "Caution: Federal law prohibits the transfer of this drug to any person other than the patient..." Other warnings depend on drug type. This notice reinforces controlled distribution laws.

Q615. Answer: B

Explanation: The subscription includes compounding or dispensing directions for the pharmacist, granting permission to prepare the drug. The superscription is the "Rx" symbol, inscription lists ingredients, and Signa gives patient directions. Understanding these sections prevents transcription errors.

Q616. Answer: C

Explanation: Powder strength and diluent volume determine the final concentration (mg/mL). The NDC or manufacturer does not affect concentration. Knowing these ensures the correct dosage per milliliter, critical for pediatric and liquid medication accuracy.

Q617. Answer: C

Explanation: Glass ampules must be drawn using filter needles to prevent glass shard contamination. Other injectable vials, like insulin or ampicillin, do not require filters. Proper technique ensures sterility and patient safety in parenteral preparation.

Q618. Answer: B

Explanation: NPO (nil per os) means "nothing by mouth." It indicates fasting before procedures or certain medication administrations. Confusing it with "do not crush" or "PRN" may lead to administration errors. Understanding medical abbreviations is critical for correct order interpretation.

Q619. Answer: A

Explanation: Patient name and date of birth uniquely identify individuals and prevent wrong-patient dispensing. BIN, DEA, or NPI relate to insurance and prescribers, not patient identity. Verifying both identifiers safeguards against one of the most common dispensing errors.

Q620. Answer: B

Explanation: Unit-dose labels contain essential product data for hospital use—drug name, strength, lot, and expiration—but exclude patient identifiers. Prescription labels include patient details, while auxiliary labels give warnings. Accurate labeling ensures traceability and proper hospital medication administration.

Q621. Answer: C

Explanation: (250 mg ÷ 5 mL) = 50 mg/mL. Then, 50 × 30 = 1500 mg total. This proportional setup ensures consistent conversion across volumes. Calculating properly avoids underdosing or overdosing, particularly in pediatric liquid preparations.

Q622. Answer: A

Explanation: Missing controlled substances must be reported on DEA Form 106 as a loss or theft. Ignoring or delaying the report violates DEA compliance. Prompt reporting ensures accountability and maintains accurate controlled substance inventory.

Q623. Answer: A

Explanation: The Desired ÷ Have × Quantity formula determines how much to dispense or use when converting between concentrations. Distractors invert relationships and yield incorrect amounts. Applying the correct ratio ensures precise compounding and dosing.

Q624. Answer: A

Explanation: "Lisinopril 10 mg #30" lacks Sig instructions (route, frequency, and dose directions). All other examples include complete Sigs. Pharmacists must contact the prescriber before filling to ensure patient safety and legal compliance.

Q625. Answer: B

Explanation: Antibiotic suspensions such as amoxicillin require refrigeration and shaking to maintain potency and uniform dosing. "Dizziness" applies to sedatives, and "milk" or "empty stomach" vary by medication. Correct auxiliary labels prevent degradation and promote patient compliance.

Q626. Answer: C

Explanation: Two doses of 50 mg each equal 100 mg total daily. Misreading BID as once daily halves the intended dose. Understanding standard dosing frequency abbreviations prevents therapeutic failure or toxicity.

Q627. Answer: C

Explanation: Technicians may enter and verify prescription data but cannot counsel, change therapy, or approve substitutions—those are pharmacist-only duties. Following scope of practice ensures legal compliance and patient safety in pharmacy operations.

Q628. Answer: B

Explanation: "TID" means ter in die, or three times daily. Confusing it with "BID" (twice daily) or "QID" (four times daily) can cause under- or overdosing. Recognizing standard medical abbreviations ensures precise interpretation and accurate medication labeling during order entry.

Q629. Answer: C

Explanation: When a drug interaction alert appears, the technician must notify the pharmacist immediately. Only pharmacists can assess clinical significance. Ignoring or overriding alerts without review endangers patient safety. Proper escalation ensures safe, compliant dispensing practices.

Q630. Answer: B

Explanation: Counting trays and spatulas maintain hygiene and accuracy while preventing cross-contamination. Counting by hand or visually estimating is unsafe and prone to error. Using proper equipment is a standard of practice in pharmacy dispensing workflow.

Q631. Answer: B

Explanation: The SIG line communicates the prescriber's directions for patient use—dose, route, frequency, and duration. It ensures patients take medications correctly. Other data like expiration or manufacturer are listed elsewhere. Accurate transcription of the SIG promotes adherence and safety.

Q632. Answer: B

Explanation: One tablespoon equals 15 mL. One teaspoon equals 5 mL, and one ounce equals approximately 30 mL. Remembering accurate conversions prevents incorrect compounding and dosage calculations, both critical for safe medication preparation and dispensing.

Q633. Answer: C

Explanation: Drug Facts and Comparisons provides comprehensive listings of brand and generic drug names, formulations, and strengths—ideal for spelling verification. The DEA and FDA resources focus on regulation, not drug spelling. Accurate reference use prevents wrong-drug entry errors.

Q634. Answer: B

Explanation: Duplicate therapy alerts must be reviewed by a pharmacist to decide clinical appropriateness. Technicians cannot discontinue medications. Duplicate alerts signal overlapping drug classes that may cause toxicity or inefficacy. Escalating to the pharmacist ensures proper clinical judgment.

Q635. Answer: A
Explanation: BIN, PCN, and ID numbers route insurance claims correctly. Errors in these fields cause rejections or billing delays. NDC codes affect product identification but not claim routing. Verifying payer data maintains workflow efficiency and reimbursement accuracy.
Q636. Answer: B
Explanation: A beyond-use date (BUD) indicates how long a compounded preparation remains stable. Manufacturer lot numbers are used only for manufactured products. Including BUDs complies with USP <795>/<797> standards and prevents the use of expired compounded products.
Q637. Answer: A
Explanation: Schedule II medications (e.g., oxycodone) cannot be refilled or transferred; each fill requires a new prescription. Schedules III–V allow limited refills. Knowing schedule restrictions ensures compliance with DEA regulations and prevents legal violations.
Q638. Answer: C
Explanation: Any unusual or excessive dose must be reported to the pharmacist for review. Technicians cannot alter or assume intent. Reporting suspected calculation errors prevents overdosing and maintains safety protocols.
Q639. Answer: A
Explanation: DAW means "Dispense as written," indicating no generic substitution allowed. "Dispense at will" or similar meanings are incorrect. Technicians must enter DAW codes accurately to comply with payer rules and prescriber intent.
Q640. Answer: C
Explanation: Divide total volume by rate: $500 \div 125 = 4$ hours. Knowing basic IV flow calculations ensures accurate timing for patient infusions and prevents under- or over-infusion errors in order processing.
Q641. Answer: C
Explanation: Pharmacists must clarify illegible prescriptions directly with the prescriber. Technicians cannot interpret or assume unclear instructions. Skipping directions compromises safety. Proper verification ensures accuracy and legal compliance.
Q642. Answer: A
Explanation: During restocking, technicians should record lot numbers and expiration dates to maintain traceability and facilitate recalls. Repackaging or altering labels are pharmacist or manufacturer responsibilities. Accurate recordkeeping ensures inventory integrity.
Q643. Answer: A
Explanation: The inscription lists the medication's name, strength, and ingredients. The superscription is the "Rx" symbol, subscription contains compounding directions, and Signa provides patient instructions. Recognizing parts of a prescription aids accurate transcription and labeling.
Q644. Answer: B
Explanation: Expired drugs must be quarantined and clearly separated to prevent accidental dispensing. They cannot be sold or transferred once past expiration. Segregating ensures compliance with FDA and state regulations.
Q645. Answer: C
Explanation: A STAT order requires immediate single administration for urgent treatment. Standing and routine orders involve scheduled doses, while PRN orders are as needed. Understanding order types ensures proper processing and prioritization in institutional settings.
Q646. Answer: C
Explanation: $24 \div 4 = 6$ doses per day $\times$ 10 mg = 60 mg total. Verifying cumulative dose prevents toxicity and helps track narcotic usage. Dosage calculation accuracy is essential in parenteral order entry.
Q647. Answer: B

Explanation: The pharmacist's final check ensures the medication, directions, and patient details are correct and that the prescription meets legal requirements. Technicians prepare and enter data, but pharmacists perform the clinical and legal verification before release.

Q648. Answer: B

Explanation: Reading back and verifying the entry with the original order ensures accuracy. Auto-fill and multitasking increase the risk of data errors. Careful, single-entry verification minimizes transcription mistakes and improves patient safety during order processing.

Q649. Answer: A

Explanation: "PC" stands for post cibum, meaning "after meals." It is often paired with medications requiring food to avoid stomach irritation. Confusing "PC" with "AC" (before meals) alters drug absorption timing. Recognizing medical abbreviations ensures accurate labeling and patient compliance.

Q650. Answer: D

Explanation: 10 mL per dose × 3 doses daily × 10 days = 300 mL total. Accurate multiplication prevents underfilling and ensures full therapy duration. Calculating quantity correctly supports effective treatment and minimizes refill interruptions.

Made in United States
Orlando, FL
04 November 2026

90201062R00087